Research Ethics Forum

Volume 9

This Series, Research Ethics Forum, aims to encourage discussion in the field of research ethics and the ethics of research. Volumes included can range from foundational issues to practical issues in research ethics. No disciplinary lines or borders are drawn and submissions are welcome from all disciplines as well as scholars from around the world. We are particularly interested in texts addressing neglected topics in research ethics, as well as those which challenge common practices and beliefs about research ethics. By means of this Series we aim to contribute to the ever important dialogue concerning the ethics of how research is conducted nationally and internationally. Possible topics include: Research Ethics Committees, Clinical trials, International research ethics regulations, Informed consent, Risk-benefit calculations, Conflicts of interest, Industry-funded research, Exploitation, Qualitative research ethics, Social science research ethics, Ghostwriting, Bias, Animal research, Research participants.

Dónal O'Mathúna · Ron Iphofen
Editors

Ethics, Integrity and Policymaking

The Value of the Case Study

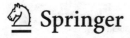 Springer

Editors
Dónal O'Mathúna
College of Nursing
The Ohio State University
Columbus, OH, USA

Ron Iphofen
Independent Researcher
La Rochelle, France

ISSN 2212-9529 ISSN 2212-9537 (electronic)
Research Ethics Forum
ISBN 978-3-031-15748-6 ISBN 978-3-031-15746-2 (eBook)
https://doi.org/10.1007/978-3-031-15746-2

This Springer imprint is published by the registered company Springer Nature Switzerland AG
The registered company address is: Gewerbestrasse 11, 6330 Cham, Switzerland

Acknowledgements

This open access volume was made possible and funded by the EU-funded PRO-RES Project. PRO-RES is a European Commission-funded project aiming to PROmote ethics and integrity in non-medical RESearch by building an evidence-supported guidance framework for all non-medical sciences and humanities disciplines adopting social science methodologies (https://prores-project.eu/). The project has developed the STEP (Scientific, Trustworthy and Ethical evidence for Policy) ACCORD which interested stakeholders are invited to consider and sign (https://pro res-project.eu/#Accord). The PRO-RES project received funding from the European Union's Horizon 2020 research and innovation programme under Grant Agreement No. 788352. The editors are consortium partners and the authors for the chapters include consortium partners and other stakeholders committed to the aims of the project—including other consortium partners. The editors wish to express their gratitude for the care and commitment demonstrated by the authors to this collection in addressing the sensitive and complex ethical issues raised in this research arena.

Contents

Chapter 1
Making a Case for the Case: An Introduction

Dónal O'Mathúna and Ron Iphofen

Abstract This chapter agues for the importance of case studies in generating evidence to guide and/or support policymaking across a variety of fields. Case studies can offer the kind of depth and detail vital to the nuances of context, which may be important in securing effective policies that take account of influences not easily identified in more generalised studies. Case studies can be written in a variety of ways which are overviewed in this chapter, and can also be written with different purposes in mind. At the same time, case studies have limitations, particularly when evidence of causation is sought. Understanding these can help to ensure that case studies are appropriately used to assist in policymaking. This chapter also provides an overview of the types of case studies found in the rest of this volume, and briefly summarises the themes and topics addressed in each of the other chapters.

Keywords Case study · Ethics · Research · Evidence · Policymaking · Context

1.1 Judging the Ethics of Research

When asked to judge the ethical issues involved in research or any evidence-gathering activity, any research ethicist worth their salt will (or should) reply, at least initially: 'It depends'. This is neither sophistry nor evasive legalism. Instead, it is a specific form of casuistry used in ethics in which general ethical principles are applied to the specifics of actual cases and inferences made through analogy. It is valued as a structured yet flexible approach to real-world ethical challenges. Case study methods recognise the complexities of depth and detail involved in assessing research activities. Another way of putting this is to say: 'Don't ask me to make a judgement about a piece of research until I have the details of the project and the context in which it will or did take place.' Understanding and fully explicating a context is vital as far as ethical

D. O'Mathúna (✉)
College of Nursing and Center for Bioethics, The Ohio State University, Columbus, OH, USA
e-mail: omathuna.6@osu.edu

R. Iphofen
Independent Research Consultant, La Rochelle, France

© The Author(s) 2022   1
D. O'Mathúna and R. Iphofen (eds.), *Ethics, Integrity and Policymaking*, Research Ethics
Forum 9, https://doi.org/10.1007/978-3-031-15746-2_1

research (and evidence-gathering) is concerned, along with taking account of the complex interrelationship between context and method (Miller and Dingwall 1997).

This rationale lies behind this collection of case studies which is one outcome from the EU-funded PRO-RES Project.[1] One aim of this project was to establish the virtues, values, principles and standards most commonly held as supportive of ethical practice by researchers, scientists and evidence-generators and users. The project team conducted desk research, workshops and consulted throughout the project with a wide range of stakeholders (PRO-RES 2021a). The resulting Scientific, Trustworthy, and Ethical evidence for Policy (STEP) ACCORD was devised, which all stakeholders could sign up to and endorse in the interests of ensuring any policies which are the outcome of research findings are based upon ethical evidence (PRO-RES 2021b).

By 'ethical evidence' we mean results and findings that have been generated by research and other activities during which the standards of research ethics and integrity have been upheld (Iphofen and O'Mathúna 2022). The first statement of the STEP ACCORD is that policy should be evidence-based, meaning that it is underpinned by high-quality research, analysis and evidence (PRO-RES 2021b). While our topic could be said to be research ethics, we have chosen to refer more broadly to *evidence-generating* activities. Much debate has occurred over the precise definition of research under the apparent assumption that 'non-research projects' fall outside the purview of requirements to obtain ethics approval from an ethics review body. This debate is more about the regulation of research than the ethics of research and has contributed to an unbalanced approach to the ethics of research (O'Mathúna 2018). Research and evidence-generating activities raise many ethical concerns, some similar and some distinct. When the focus is primarily on which projects need to obtain what sort of ethics approval from which type of committee, the ethical issues raised by those activities themselves can receive insufficient attention. This can leave everyone involved with these activities either struggling to figure out how to manage complex and challenging ethical dilemmas or pushing ahead with those activities confident that their approval letter means they have fulfilled all their ethical responsibilities. Unfortunately, this can lead to a view that research ethics is an impediment and burden that must be overcome so that the important work in the research itself can get going.

The alternative perspective advocated by PRO-RES, and the authors of the chapters in this volume, is that ethics underpins all phases of research, from when the idea for a project is conceived, all the way through its design and implementation, and on to how its findings are disseminated and put into practice in individual decisions or in policy. Given the range of activities involved in all these phases, multiple types of ethical issues can arise. Each occurs in its own context of time and place, and this must be taken into account. While ethical principles and theories have important

---

[1] PRO-RES is a European Commission-funded project aiming to *PROmote ethics and integrity in non-medical RESearch* by building a supported guidance framework for all non-medical sciences and humanities disciplines adopting social science methodologies. This project has received funding from the European Union's Horizon 2020 research and innovation programme under grant agreement No 788352. Open access fees for this volume were paid for through the PRO-RES funding.

contributions to make at each of these points, case studies are also very important. These allow for the normative effects of various assumptions and declarations to be judged in context. We therefore asked the authors of this volume's chapters to identify various case studies which would demonstrate the ethical challenges entailed in various types of research and evidence-generating activities. These illustrative case studies explore various innovative topics and fields that raise challenges requiring ethical reflection and careful policymaking responses. The cases highlight diverse ethical issues and provide lessons for the various options available for policymaking (see Sect. 1.6. below). Cases are drawn from many fields, including artificial intelligence, space science, energy, data protection, professional research practice and pandemic planning. The issues are examined in different locations, including Europe, India, Africa and in global contexts. Each case is examined in detail and also helps to anticipate lessons that could be learned and applied in other situations where ethical evidence is needed to inform evidence-based policymaking.

1.2 The Case for Cases

Case studies have increasingly been used, particularly in social science (Exworthy and Powell 2012). Many reasons underlie this trend, one being the movement towards evidence-based practice. Case studies provide a methodology by which a detailed study can be conducted of a social unit, whether that unit is a person, an organization, a policy or a larger group or system (Exworthy and Powell 2012). The case study is amenable to various methodologies, mostly qualitative, which allow investigations via documentary analyses, interviews, focus groups, observations, and more.

At the same time, consensus is lacking over the precise nature of a case study. Various definitions have been offered, but Yin (2017) provides a widely cited definition with two parts. One is that a case study is an in-depth inquiry into a real-life phenomenon where the context is highly pertinent. The second part of Yin's definition addresses the many variables involved in the case, the multiple sources of evidence explored, and the inclusion of theoretical propositions to guide the analysis. While Yin's emphasis is on the case study as a research method, he identifies important elements of broader relevance that point to the particular value of the case study for examining ethical issues.

Other definitions of case studies emphasize their story or narrative aspects (Gwee 2018). These stories frequently highlight a dilemma in contextually rich ways, with an emphasis on how decisions can be or need to be made. Case studies are particularly helpful with ethical issues to provide crucial context and explore (and evaluate) how ethical decisions have been made or need to be made. Classic cases include the Tuskegee public health syphilis study, the Henrietta Lacks human cell line case, the Milgram and Zimbardo psychology cases, the Tea Room Trade case, and the Belfast Project in oral history research (examined here in Chap. 10). Cases exemplify core ethical principles, and how they were applied or misapplied; in addition, they examine how policies have worked well or not (Chaps. 2, 3 and 5). Cases can examine ethics in long-standing issues (like research misconduct (Chap. 7), energy production (Chap. 8), or Chap. 11's consideration of researchers breaking the law), or with innovations in need of further ethical reflection because of their novelty (like extended space flight (Chap. 9) and AI (Chaps. 13 and 14), with the latter looking at automation in legal systems). These case studies help to situate the innovations within the context of widely regarded ethical principles and theories, and allow comparisons to be made with other technologies or practices where ethical positions have been developed. In doing so, these case studies offer pointers and suggestions for policymakers given that they are the ones who will develop applicable policies.

1.3   Research Design and Causal Inference

Not everyone is convinced of the value of the case study. It must be admitted that they have limitations, which we will reflect on shortly. Yet we believe that others go too far in their criticisms, revealing instead some prejudices against the value of the case (Yin 2017). In what has become a classic text for research design, Campbell and Stanley (1963) have few good words for what they call the 'One Shot Case Study.' They rank it below two other 'pre-experimental' designs—the One-Group Pretest–Posttest and the Static-Group Comparison—and conclude that case studies "have such a total absence of control to be of almost no scientific value" (Campbell and Stanley 1963, 6). The other designs have, in turn, a baseline and outcome measure and some degree of comparative analysis which provides them some validity. Such a criticism is legitimate if one prioritises the experimental method as the most superior in terms of effectiveness evidence and, as for Campbell and Stanley, one is striving to assess the effectiveness of educational interventions.

What is missing from that assessment is that different methodologies are more appropriate for different kinds of questions. Questions of causation and whether a particular treatment, policy or educational strategy is more effective than another are best answered by experimental methods. While experimental designs are better suited to explore causal relationships, case studies are more suited to explore "how" and "why" questions (Yin 2017). It can be more productive to view different methodologies as complementing one another, rather than examining them in hierarchical terms.

The case study approach draws on a long tradition in ethnography and anthropology: "It stresses the importance of holistic perspectives and so has more of a 'humanistic' emphasis. It recognises that there are multiple influences on any single individual or group and that most other methods neglect the thorough understanding of this range of influences. They usually focus on a chosen variable or variables which are tested in terms of their influence. A case study tends to make no initial assumptions about which are the key variables—preferring to allow the case to 'speak for itself'" (Iphofen et al. 2009, 275). This tradition has sometimes discouraged people from conducting or using case studies on the assumption that they take massive amounts of time and lead to huge reports. This is the case with ethnography, but the case study method can be applied in more limited settings and can lead to high-quality, concise reports.

Another criticism of case studies is that they cannot be used to make generalizations. Certainly, there are limits to their generalisability, but the same is true of experimental studies. One randomized controlled trial cannot be generalised to the whole population without ensuring that its details are evaluated in the context of how it was conducted.

Similarly, it should not be assumed that generalisability can adequately guide practice or policy when it comes to the specifics of an individual case. A case study should not be used to support statistical generalizations (that the same percentage found in the case will be found in the general public). But a case study can be used to expand and generalize theories and thus have much usefulness. It affords a method of examining the specific (complex) interactions occurring in a case which can only be known from the details. Such an analysis can be carried out for individuals, policies or interventions.

The current COVID-19 pandemic demonstrates the dangers of generalising in the wrong context. Some people have very mild cases of COVID-19 or are asymptomatic. Others get seriously ill and even die. Sometimes people generalise from cases they know and assume they will have mild symptoms. Then they refuse to take the COVID-19 vaccine, basically generalising from similar cases. Mass vaccination is recommended for the sake of the health of the public (generalised health) and to limit the spread of a deadly virus. Cases are reported of people having adverse reactions to COVID-19 vaccines, and some people generalise from these that they will not take whatever risks might be involved in receiving the vaccine themselves. It might be theoretically possible to discover which individuals WILL react adversely to immunisation on a population level. But it is highly complex and expensive to do so, and takes an extensive period of time. Given the urgency of benefitting the health of 'the public', policymakers have decided that the risks to a sub-group are warranted. Only after the emergence of epidemiological data disclosing negative effects of *some* vaccines on *some* individuals will it become more clear which characteristics typify those cases which are likely to experience the adverse effects, and more accurately quantify the risks of experiencing those effects.

Much literature now points to the advantages and disadvantages of case studies (Gomm et al. 2000), and how to use them and conduct them with adequate rigour to ensure the validity of the evidence generated (Schell 1992; Yin 2011, 2017). At the same time, legitimate critiques have been made of some case studies because they have been conducted without adequate rigor, in unsystematic ways, or in ways that allowed bias to have more influence than evidence (Hammersley 2001). Part of the problem here is similar to interviewing, where some will assume that since interviews are a form of conversation, anyone can do it. Case studies have some similarities to stories, but that doesn't mean they are quick and easy ways to report on events. That view can lead to the situation where "most people feel that they can prepare a case study, and nearly all of us believe we can understand one. Since neither view is well founded, the case study receives a lot of approbation it does not deserve" (Hoaglin et al., cited in Yin 2017, 16).

Case studies can be conducted and used in a wide range of ways (Gwee 2018). Case studies can be used as a research method, as a teaching tool, as a way of recording events so that learning can be applied to practice, and to facilitate practical problem-solving skills (Luck et al. 2006). Significant differences exist between a case study that was developed and used in research compared to one used for teaching (Yin 2017). A valid rationale for studying a 'case' should be provided so that it is clear that the proposed method is suitable to the topic and subject being studied. The unit of study for a case could be an individual person, social group, community, or society. Sometimes that specific case alone will constitute the actual research project. Thus, the study could be of one individual's experience, with insights and understanding gained of the individual's situation which could be of use to understand others' experiences. Often there will be attempts made at a comparison between cases—one organisation being compared to another, with both being studied in some detail, and in terms of the same or similar criteria. Given this variety, it is important to use cases in ways appropriate to how they were generated.

The case study continues to be an important piece of evidence in clinical decision-making in medicine and healthcare. Here, case studies do not demonstrate causation or effectiveness, but are used as an important step in understanding the experiences of patients, particularly with a new or confusing set of symptoms. This was clearly seen as clinicians published case studies describing a new respiratory infection which the world now knows to be COVID-19. Only as case studies were generated, and the patterns brought together in larger collections of cases, did the characteristics of the illness come to inform those seeking to diagnose at the bedside (Borges do Nascimento et al. 2020). Indeed case studies are frequently favoured in nursing, healthcare and social work research where professional missions require a focus on the care of the individual and where cases facilitate making use of the range of research paradigms (Galatzer-Levy et al. 2000; Mattaini 1996; Gray 1998; Luck et al. 2006).

1.4 Devil's in the Detail

Our main concern in this collection is not with case study aetiology but rather to draw on the advantages of the method to highlight key ethical issues related to the use of evidence in influencing policy. Thus, we make no claim to causal 'generalisation' on the basis of these reports—but instead we seek to help elucidate ethics issues, if even theoretical, and anticipate responses and obstacles in similar situations and contexts that might help decision-making in novel circumstances. A key strength of case studies is their capacity to connect abstract theoretical concepts to the complex realities of practice and the real world (Luck et al. 2006). Ethics cases clearly fit this description and allow the contextual details of issues and dilemmas to be included in discussions of how ethical principles apply as policy is being developed.

Since cases are highly focussed on the specifics of the situation, more time can be given over to data gathering which may be of both qualitative and quantitative natures. Given the many variables involved in the 'real life' setting, increased methodological flexibility is required (Yin 2017). This means seeking to maximise the data sources—such as archives (personal and public), records (such as personal diaries), observations (participant and covert) and interviews (face-to-face and online)—and revisiting all sources when necessary and as case participants and time allows.

1.5 Cases and Policymaking

Case studies allow researchers and practitioners to learn from the specifics of a situation and apply that learning in similar situations. Ethics case studies allow such reflection to facilitate the development of ethical decision-making skills. This volume has major interests in ethics and evidence-generation (research), but also in a third area: policymaking. Cases can influence policymaking, such as how one case can receive widespread attention and become the impetus to create policy that aims to prevent similar cases. For example, the US federal Brady Law was enacted in 1993 to require background checks on people before they purchase a gun (ATF 2021). The law was named for White House Press Secretary James Brady, and his case became widely known in the US. He was shot and paralyzed during John Hinckley, Jr.'s 1981 assassination attempt on President Ronald Reagan. Another example, this time in a research context, was how the Tuskegee Syphilis Study led, after its public exposure in 1971, to the US Department of Health, Education and Welfare appointing an expert panel to examine the ethics of that case. This resulted in federal policymakers enacting the National Research Act in 1974, which included setting up a national commission that published the Belmont Report in 1976. This report continues to strongly influence research ethics practice around the world. These examples highlight the power of a case study to influence policymaking.

One of the challenges for policymakers, though, is that compelling cases can often be provided for opposite sides of an issue. Also, while the Belmont Report has been praised for articulating a small number of key ethical principles, how those principles should be applied in specific instances of research remains an ongoing challenge and a point of much discussion. This is particularly relevant for innovative techniques and technologies. Hence the importance of cases interacting with general principles and leading to ongoing reflection and debate over the applicable cases. At the same time, new areas of research and evidence generation activities will lead to questions about how existing ethical principles and values apply. New case studies can help to facilitate that reflection, which can then allow policymakers to consider whether existing policy should be adapted or whether whole new areas of policy are needed.

Case studies also can play an important role in learning from and evaluating policy. Policymakers tend to focus on practical, day-to-day concerns and with the introduction of new programmes (Exworthy and Peckam 2012). Time and resources may be scant when it comes to evaluating how well existing policies are performing or reflecting on how policies can be adapted to overcome shortcomings (Hunter 2003). Effective policies may exist elsewhere (historically or geographically) and be more easily adapted to a new context instead of starting policymaking from scratch. Case studies can permit learning from past policies (or situations where policies did not exist), and they can illuminate various factors that should be explored in more detail in the context of the current issue or situation. Chaps. 2, 3 and 5 in this volume are examples of this type of case study.

1.6   The Moral Gain

This volume reflects the ambiguity of ethical dilemmas in contemporary policy-making. Analyses will reflect current debates where consensus has not been achieved yet. These cases illustrate key points made throughout the PRO-RES project: that ethical decision-making is a fluid enterprise, where values, principles and standards must constantly be applied to new situations, new events and new research developments. The cases illustrate how no 'one point' exists in the research process where judgements about ethics can be regarded as 'final.' Case studies provide excellent ways for readers to develop important decision-making skills.

Research produces novel products and processes which can have broad implications for society, the environment and relationships. Research methods themselves are modified or applied in new ways and places, requiring further ethical reflection. New topics and whole fields of research develop and require careful evaluation and thoughtful responses. New case studies are needed because research constantly generates new issues and new ethics questions for policymaking.

The cases found in this volume address a wide range of topics and involve several disciplines. The cases were selected by the parameters of the PRO-RES project and the Horizon 2020 funding call to which it responded. First, the call was concerned with both research ethics and scientific integrity and each of the cases addresses one or both of these areas. The call sought projects that addressed non-medical research, and the cases here address disciplines such as social sciences, engineering, artificial intelligence and One Health. The call also sought particular attention be given to (a) covert research, (b) working in dangerous areas/conflict zones and (c) behavioral research collecting data from social media/internet sources. Hence, we included cases that addressed each of these areas. Finally, while an EU-funded project can be expected to have a European focus, the issues addressed have global implications. Therefore, we wanted to include cases studies from outside Europe and did so by involving authors from India and Africa to reflect on the volume's areas of interest.

The first case study offered in this volume (Chap. 2) examines a significant policy approach taken by the European Union to address ethics and integrity in research and innovation: Responsible Research and Innovation (RRI). This chapter examines the lessons that can be learned from RRI in a European context. Chapter 3 elaborates on this topic with another policy learning case study, but this time examining RRI in India. One of the critiques made of RRI is that it can be Euro-centric. This case study examines this claim, and also describes how a distinctively Indian concept, Scientific Temper, can add to and contextualise RRI. Chapter 4 takes a different approach in being a case study of the development of research ethics guidance in the United Kingdom (UK). It explores the history underlying the research ethics framework commissioned by the UK Research Integrity Office (UKRIO) and the Association of Research Managers and Administrators (ARMA), and points to lessons that can be learned about the policy-development process itself.

While staying focused on policy related to research ethics, the chapters that follow include case studies that address more targeted concerns. Chapter 5 examines the impact of the European Union's (EU) General Data Protection Regulation (GDPR) in the Republic of Croatia. Research data collected in Croatia is used to explore the handling of personal data before and after the introduction of GDPR. This case study aims to provide lessons learned that could contribute to research ethics policies and procedures in other European Member States.

Chapter 6 moves from policy itself to the role of policy advisors in policymaking. This case study explores the distinct responsibilities of those elevated to the role of "policy advisor," especially given the current lack of policy to regulate this field or how its advice is used by policymakers. Next, Chap. 7 straddles the previous chapters' focus on policy and its evaluation while introducing the focus of the next section on historical case studies. This chapter uses the so-called "race for the superconductor" as a case study by which the PRO-RES ethics framework is used to explore specific ethical dilemmas (PRO-RES 2021b). This case study is especially useful for policymakers because of how it reveals the multiple difficulties in balancing economic, political, institutional and professional requirements and values.

The next case study continues the use of historical cases, but here to explore the challenges facing innovative research into unorthodox energy technology that has the potential to displace traditional energy suppliers. The wave power case in Chap. 8 highlights how conducting research with integrity can have serious consequences and come with considerable cost. The case also points to the importance of transparency in how evidence is used in policymaking so that trust in science and scientists is promoted at the same time as science is used in the public interest. Another area of cutting-edge scientific innovation is explored in Chap. 9, but this time looking to the future. This case study examines space exploration, and specifically the ethical issues around establishing safe exposure standards for astronauts embarking on extended duration spaceflights. This case highlights the ethical challenges in policymaking focused on an elite group of people (astronauts) who embark on extremely risky activities in the name of science and humanity.

Chapter 10 moves from the physical sciences to the social sciences. The Belfast Project provides a case study to explore the ethical challenges of conducting research after violent conflict. In this case, researchers promised anonymity and confidentiality to research participants, yet that was overturned through legal proceedings which highlighted the limits of confidentiality in research. This case points to the difficulty of balancing the value of research archives in understanding conflict against the value of providing juridical evidence to promote justice. Another social science case is examined in Chap. 11, this time in ethnography. This so-called 'urban explorer' case study explores the justifications that might exist for undertaking covert research where researchers break the law (in this case by trespassing) in order to investigate a topic that would remain otherwise poorly understood. This case raises a number of important questions for policymakers around: the freedoms that researchers should be given to act in the public interest; when researchers are justified in breaking the law; and what responsibilities and consequences researchers should accept if they believe they are justified in doing so.

Further complexity in research and evidence generation is introduced in Chap. 12. A case study in *One Health* is used to explore ethical issues at the intersection of animal, human and environmental ethics. The pertinence of such studies has been highlighted by COVID-19, yet policies lag behind in recognising the urgency and complexity of initiating investigations into novel outbreaks, such as the one discussed here that occurred among animals in Ethiopia. Chapter 13 retains the COVID-19 setting, but returns the attention to technological innovation. Artificial intelligence (AI) is the focus of these two chapters in the volume, here examining the ethical challenges arising from the emergency authorisation of using AI to respond to the public health needs created by the COVID-19 pandemic. Chapter 14 addresses a longer term use of AI in addressing problems and challenges in the legal system. Using the so-called Robodebt case, the chapter explores the reasons why legal systems are turning to AI and other automated procedures. The Robodebt case highlights problems when AI algorithms are built on inaccurate assumptions and implemented with little human oversight. This case shows the massive problems for hundreds of thousands of Australians who became victims of poorly conceived AI and makes recommendations to assist policymakers to avoid similar debacles. The last chapter (Chap. 15) draws some general conclusions from all the cases that are relevant when using case studies.

1.7   Into the Future

This volume focuses on ethics in research and professional integrity and how we can be clear about the lessons that can be drawn to assist policymakers. The cases provided cover a wide range of situations, settings, and disciplines. They cover international, national, organisational, group and individual levels of concern. Each case raises distinct issues, yet also points to some general features of research, evidence-generation, ethics and policymaking. All the studies illustrate the difficulties of drawing clear 'boundaries' between the research and the context. All these case studies show how in real situations dynamic judgements have to be made about many different issues. Guidelines and policies do help and are needed. But at the same time, researchers, policymakers and everyone else involved in evidence generation and evidence implementation need to embody the virtues that are central to good research. Judgments will need to be made in many areas, for example, about how much transparency can be allowed, or is ethically justified; how much risk can be taken, both with participants' safety and also with the researchers' safety; how much information can be disclosed to or withheld from participants in their own interests and for the benefit of the 'science'; and many others. All of these point to just how difficult it can be to apply common standards across disciplines, professions, cultures and countries. That difficulty must be acknowledged and lead to open discussions with the aim of improving practice. The cases presented here point to efforts that have been made towards this. None of them is perfect. Lessons must be learned from all of them, towards which Chap. 15 aims to be a starting point. Only by openly discussing and reflecting on past practice can lessons be learned that can inform policymaking that aims to improve future practice. In this way, ethical progress can become an essential aspect of innovation in research and evidence-generation.

References

ATF (Bureau of Alcohol, Tobacco, Firearms and Explosives). 2021. Brady law. https://www.atf. gov/rules-and-regulations/brady-law. Accessed 1 Jan 2022.

Borges do Nascimento, Israel J., Thilo C. von Groote, Dónal P. O'Mathúna, Hebatullah M. Abdulazeem, Catherine Henderson, Umesh Jayarajah, et al. 2020. Clinical, laboratory and radiological characteristics and outcomes of novel coronavirus (SARS-CoV-2) infection in humans: a systematic review and series of meta-analyses. PLoS ONE 15(9):e0239235. https://doi.org/10.1371/jou rnal.pone.0239235.

Campbell, D.T., and J.C. Stanley. 1963. *Experimental and quasi-experimental designs for research.* Chicago: Rand McNally and Company.

Exworthy, Mark, and Stephen Peckam. 2012. Policy learning from case studies in health policy. taking forward the debate. In *Shaping health policy: case study methods and analysis,* ed. Mark Exworthy, Stephen Peckham, Martin Powell, and Alison Hann, 313–328. Bristol, UK: Policy Press.

Exworthy, Mark, and Martin Powell. 2012. Case studies in health policy: an introduction. In *Shaping health policy: case study methods and analysis,* ed. Mark Exworthy, Stephen Peckham, Martin Powell, and Alison Hann, 3–20. Bristol, UK: Policy Press.

Galatzer-Levy, R.M., Bachrach, H., Skolnikoff, A., and Wadlron, S. Jr. 2000. The single case method. In *Does Psychoanalysis Work?,* 230–242. New Haven and London: Yale University Press.

Gomm, R., M. Hammersley, and P. Foster, eds. 2000. *Case study method: Key issues, key texts.* London: Sage.

Gray, M. 1998. Introducing single case study research design: an overview. *Nurse Researcher* 5 (4): 15–24.

Gwee, June. 2018. *The case writer's toolkit.* Singapore: Palgrave Macmillan.

Hammersley, M. 2001. Which side was Becker on? Questioning political and epistemological radicalism. *Qualitative Research* 1 (1): 91–110.

Hunter, D.J. 2003. Evidence-based policy and practice: riding for a fall? *Journal of the Royal Society of Medicine* 96 (4): 194–196. https://www.ncbi.nlm.nih.gov/pmc/articles/PMC539453/

Iphofen, R., and D. O'Mathúna (eds.). 2022. *Ethical evidence and policymaking: interdisciplinary and international research.* Bristol, UK: Policy Press.

Iphofen, R., A. Krayer, and C.A. Robinson. 2009. *Reviewing and reading social care research: from ideas to findings.* Bangor: Bangor University.

Luck, L., D. Jackson, and K. Usher. 2006. Case study: a bridge across the paradigms. *Nursing Inquiry* 13 (2): 103–109.

Mattaini, M.A. 1996. The abuse and neglect of single-case designs. *Research on Social Work Practice* 6 (1): 83–90.

Miller, G., and R. Dingwall. 1997. *Context and method in qualitative research.* London: Sage.

O'Mathúna, Dónal. 2018. The dual imperative in disaster research ethics. In *SAGE Handbook of qualitative research ethics,* ed. Ron Iphofen and Martin Tolich, 441–454. London: SAGE.

PRO-RES. 2021a. The foundational statements for ethical research. http://prores-project.eu/the-fou ndational-statements-for-ethical-research-practice/. Accessed 1 Jan 2022.

PRO-RES. 2021b. Accord. https://prores-project.eu/#Accord. Accessed 1 Jan 2022.

Schell, C. 1992. *The Value of the Case Study as a Research Strategy*. Manchester Business School.

Yin, Robert K. 2011. *Applications of case study research*, 3rd ed. London: Sage.

Yin, Robert K. 2017. *Case study research and applications: design and methods*, 6th ed. London: Sage.

Chapter 2
Responsible Research and Innovation (RRI) and Research Ethics

Giovanna Declich, Maresa Berliri, and Alfonso Alfonsi

Abstract The case study presented in this chapter concerns the policy adopted by the European Commission for better management of the relationship between science and society, with a focus on the ethics of scientific research. This policy, since 2011, has been based on the notion of responsible research and innovation (RRI). We discuss the RRI strategy as an attempt to include ethics within a broader policy framework to respond to the challenges emerging in the European research and innovation landscape. To do so, we examine the origins of the RRI idea, its incorporation into Commission policy, as well as its effectiveness and its impacts. We further discuss whether it has served its purpose in light of the fact that the terminology associated with RRI has been progressively downplayed in more recent years. Positive impacts exist, but also difficulties as RRI aims to take root and enhance and strengthen its ethical aspects. In conclusion, some lessons learned from this ten-year policy effort are presented, exploring the potentialities and limits of such an approach for the renewal of research ethics, and discussing what can be the theoretical and practical legacy of RRI for contemporary scientific and technological innovation policies.

Keywords Responsible Research and Innovation (RRI) · Research ethics · Anticipation · Reflexivity · Inclusion · Responsiveness · Evidence-based policymaking

2.1 Introduction: RRI as a Policy Response to the Ethical Challenge of the Changing Relationship Between Science and Society

The case study examined in this chapter explores responsible research and innovation (RRI) as a European Union (EU) policy that has strong ethical motivations and implications. We consider the whole arc of the RRI approach in EU policies about

G. Declich · M. Berliri (✉) · A. Alfonsi
Knowledge and Innovation, Rome, Italy
e-mail: berliri@knowledge-innovation.org

© The Author(s) 2022
D. O'Mathúna and R. Iphofen (eds.), *Ethics, Integrity and Policymaking*, Research Ethics Forum 9, https://doi.org/10.1007/978-3-031-15746-2_2

science intended here as a case of a peculiar organised and policy-oriented reaction of the EU to the changes in scientific production and to the uncertainty this change generates in the research systems itself and in society as a whole. In a nutshell, RRI can be seen as an ambitious challenge for the formulation of research and innovation policies driven by the needs of society and engaging all societal actors via inclusive participatory approaches.

Our chapter examines the attempt made through the RRI strategy to include ethics within a broader policy framework, with the aim of responding in policy terms to the problem of the inadequacy of traditional research ethics in dealing with the challenges emerging at various levels in the European research and innovation landscape. A rapid analysis of the idea and practice of RRI is conducted to understand how best (and first of all whether) the concerns about research ethics and integrity can be incorporated into decision-making. To do so, the origins of the RRI idea, its incorporation into Commission policy, the effectiveness of the idea and its impacts are examined, and whether it has actually served its purpose is discussed, not least in light of the fact that the conceptualisation associated with RRI has been progressively downplayed in more recent years. There have been positive impacts, but also difficulties for RRI to take root and to enhance and strengthen its ethical aspects.

In the last part of the text, the lessons learnt from this ten-year policy effort are discussed, exploring the potentialities and limits of such an approach for an effective renewal of research ethics, both in theoretical terms and in terms of practices and tools, in the framework of a more general reflection on the theoretical and practical legacy of RRI for contemporary scientific and technological innovation policies.

We wish to disclose at the outset that the authors of this chapter have been and still are involved in EU-funded projects concerning RRI, both where RRI is the subject of study and where RRI is an approach proactively promoted in scientific institutions. In writing the chapter, we have tried to make use of the "insider" perspective gained through our experience, while at the same time distancing ourselves enough to provide a frank and realistic assessment of its strong points and drawbacks, and of its overall effectiveness.

2.2 The Context: The Transformations of Science and Society at the Turn of the Twentieth and Twenty-First Centuries

In order to understand the drivers that brought about RRI, it is necessary to situate them within the broader context of the transition phase that science and innovation are going through, which, in turn, is part of a broader shift from modern to post-modern society, which also affects and to some extent weakens the main social institutions of modernity.

The changes occurring in science and technology offer many new opportunities but are also exposing research organisations and researchers to tangible risks, such as diminishing authority, increasing uncertainty about procedures and standards, and/or a declining and more difficult access to resources.

Moreover, such changes have transformed the way in which research is conducted and disseminated. Research is now more open and its results more easily accessible to citizens, but at the same time, it is receiving increased public scrutiny, while public distrust and disaffection towards science appear to be on the rise (House of Lords Select Committee on Science and Technology 2000; Eurobarometer 2010 and 2013), often correlated to an equal lack of trust towards the government (Wellcome Global Monitor 2018).

The formulation and saliency of the notion of responsible research and innovation should be seen against such a background, which involves a profound restructuring of the relationship of science with the rest of society.

The term "responsible innovation" could be considered as having been introduced in Europe in its current usage in 2009 after being proposed by the Nederlandse Organisatie voor Wetenschappelijk Onderzoek (NWO), the Dutch Research Council, during a series of events and projects (Stahl 2013). However, there are several antecedents that show how such a notion had already been in circulation in the European discourse on science and innovation. For instance, the European Research Advisory Board had already published in 2005 a document in preparation for the EU FP7 on Science and Society, in which the idea of a "responsive and responsible European Science" was proposed (European Commission 2006).

Going back to the late 1980s and early 1990s, we can single out as antecedents of the issues addressed by RRI the insertion of ethical, legal, and social aspects (ELSA, in Europe) or implications (ELSI, in the USA) in the research agenda (Chadwick and Hub 2013), especially in relation to such cutting-edge research as genomics and nanotechnologies, with the launch of research programs aimed at anticipating and addressing the effects generated by the development of such research and technology fields.

A further antecedent of RRI can be found in the widespread debate on the so-called "Public Engagement with Science and Technology" (PEST) approach, based on a public dialogue with scientists about the aims, methods, and results of science (Wynne and Felt 2007; Gumeirães Pereira et al. 2013). Other precursors can be considered the reflection on technology assessment (TA) (Grundwald 2011) and, in the USA, on the responsible development (Stahl 2013) and the responsible conduct of research (RCR), the latter mainly focused on research integrity issues (Kalichman 2013).

The growing concern for gender and gender equality in science, in particular those initiatives and policies oriented at activating institutional change to promote gender equality in research institutions, such as the establishment in the USA of the ADVANCE Programme of the National Science Foundation[1], can be also considered

---

[1] Established in 2001, the NSF ADVANCE program can be considered the first national funding scheme aimed at activating institutional change processes in research organisations to favour gender equality in science and innovation.

as antecedents of the RRI strategy. To this can be added the funding schemes for structural change in the European Commission Framework Programmes[2].

Finally, even the approaches advocating open access to scientific production and promoting science education for the citizenry can be viewed among the strands of concern that converged in the conception and promotion of RRI.

RRI then appears as an approach aimed to modify the consolidated social model of producing and reproducing science—often expressed with the image of the "Ivory Tower"—towards a model for science that is fully embedded in society and strongly connected and sensitive to societal expectations, needs, worries and problems.

In this frame, responsibility is intended not only as a desired outcome of a process but also as a guiding principle that should inform all the domains of science as a social institution, its actors and its structures.

2.3 An Attempt to Enhance the Ethical Dimension of RTD: Theory and Practice of RRI

On the basis of the brief narrative of the previous paragraph, we can suggest, as also argued by Stahl (2013, 709), that Responsible Research and Innovation appears to originate and develop as an attempt to cope with the so-called grand challenges which include "questions of employment, economic wellbeing and growth, issues of social coherence, and the resilience of democratic societies, demographic developments, social innovations and other topics," thus taking on the responsibility towards the society that many see as a weakness of science and scientists. An idea of "responsibility" which, as noted by d'Andrea et al. (2017) is currently being applied to many life domains, thus generating concepts like "responsible politics", "responsible eating", "responsible consumerism", "responsible religion" or "responsible lifestyle". In this sense, RRI appears grounded in substantive social processes and "resonates with the ongoing concerns related to the role of science, particularly in society" (Rip 2016, 3).

As we have seen, RRI refers to a series of meanings that have evolved over time. It has to be noted, in this regard, that such notions are by no means exactly defined nor its contents and dimensions always consistently delimited. As a matter of fact, several definitions, which are sometimes very dissimilar from the other, have been formulated by scholars and policymakers, alternatively meaning, as highlighted by Job Timmermans and Bernd Stahl (2013): something which is external to the research and innovation process, as a governance principle (von Schomberg 2012; Owen et al. 2013); a requirement to be embodied in the research and innovation process (Geoghegan-Quinn 2012); a part of the research and innovation process or even a

---

[2] The Seventh Framework Programme and the subsequent Horizon 2020, through the SiS and the SWAFS work programmes, have included funding for gender equality action plans individual research institutions and universities.

different way to make research and innovation (Stahl 2013; the Expert Group on the State of Art in Europe on RRI 2013).

One of the definitions[3] that has gained much currency is the one provided by von Schomberg in 2011: "The process by which societal actors and innovators become mutually responsive to each other with a view to the (ethical) acceptability, sustainability and societal desirability of the innovation process and its marketable products" (von Schomberg 2011, 6). Notwithstanding this conceptual indetermination, or even thanks to its "interpretive flexibility", RRI has addressed widely felt needs in the science community and has been playing an important role in framing part of European research policies. Thus, RRI has served as an "umbrella concept" which includes and tries to coordinate different sets of drivers, by defining some general ordering principles meant to better align the research and innovation process with the needs and expectations of the whole of society.

In the case of the European Union policies, RRI started to inform the discourse on research and innovation with a series of high profile meetings, such as the Brussels workshop on "responsible research and innovation" convened in May 2011 by the Directorate-General (DG) for Research of the European Commission (EC). In the following years, the notion increasingly permeated EC science policies, and towards the end of the VII Framework Programme for Science and Technology, the Science and Society program adopted the RRI notion. Thereafter, the first calls making explicit reference to RRI started to be launched. This process culminated with the eighth Framework Programme, Horizon Europe, where RRI was included as a cross-cutting issue, and as an overarching frame for the Science with and for Society program (SwafS)[4]. In Horizon 2020, the SwafS program based, among other themes, on RRI had a budget of €462 million; received more than 2,000 proposals in its various calls; and funded around 200 projects, with around 50 in the SwafS last call (Delaney et al. 2020).

While the RRI approach was somehow being institutionalised at the European level, there was a drive to "solidify" into some actionable indications what had been so far a rather broad and open process. As Owen and his co-authors (2021) point out, this occurred mainly by the introduction of the so-called "keys": gender equality in science, open access to research data and publications, research ethics and integrity, citizen engagement, and science education, integrated in the beginning with governance as a sixth key (European Commission 2014). Those keys were included in the "Rome Declaration on RRI" (November 2014) and later on identified as the founding pillars of the RRI approach. According to Owen et al., the keys were introduced because they reflected as many action lines existing in the Science in Society program prior to the notion of RRI and were expected to support the mainstreaming of RRI in the Horizon 2020 Program. In this way, however, the dynamic process of

---

[3] An outline of the different definitions of RRI can be found in d'Andrea et al. (2017) "Report on the literature Review. FIT4RRI Deliverable D.1.1", pp. 50–51.

[4] An interesting account of and reflection on these passages can be found in the paper "An unfinished journey? Reflections on a decade of responsible research and innovation, written by three leading figures in the RRI story: Richard Owen, René Von Schomberg and Phil Macnaghten.

RRI runs the risk of becoming synonymous with the keys and being subject to a sort of "reification" (Owen et al. 2021).

In this light, some authors prefer to focus on what they consider four dimensions rather than on the RRI keys.[5] These dimensions can be seen to present in a more flexible and dynamic way the exercise of responsibility towards research and innovation (Burget et al. 2017).

– Inclusion mainly refers to the engagement of different stakeholders from the early stages of research and innovation to give voice to all the concerned interests, values, needs, and beliefs.
– Anticipation refers to the capacity of envisioning the outcomes of the processes of research and innovation and understanding how current dynamics help design the future in order to prevent risks and to lead research to desirable impacts.
– Responsiveness concerns the capacity to develop proactive management of new technologies so as to identify risks and develop an ethically adequate response. According to Burget et al. (2017), responsiveness also relates to transparency (responses should be open to public debate) and accessibility (scientific results about risks and responses should be openly accessible to everyone).
– Reflexivity is mainly seen as the capacity of the research system to keep control of its own activities and assumptions, to be aware of the limits of the knowledge produced as well as to reflect on values and beliefs connected with research and innovation. Reflexivity is linked to public dialogue and collaborative approaches in science.

With the arrival of the new Framework Programme, Horizon Europe, RRI remains an operational objective of the Strategic Programme, but its visibility and also its strategic placement are reduced if compared with its role in Horizon 2020. The new program has the notions of Open Science and mission-driven innovation as its strategic drive.

This tendency to attenuate the impact of RRI is further corroborated by the answers of a panel of experts and stakeholders interviewed during a round of consultation in Summer-Fall 2020 in the framework of the Project PRO-RES[6]. Notwithstanding the fact that all the interviewees were active, in various forms, in the European research area, almost one third of them were not aware of RRI contents and objectives or showed only a very superficial knowledge thereof. Other interviewees argued that such a notion was too wide and subject to different interpretations, so generating confusion and less impact than expected for ethical aspects. Those who thought that referring to RRI could be useful for reinforcing the ethical dimensions of science tended to do so in an instrumental perspective, such as leveraging the "brand RRI" for reaching a larger audience or addressing the younger generations of scientists

---

[5] Also the dimensions of RRI can be defined in different manners. See among other Owen et al. (2012); Stilgoe et al. (2013); Lubberink et al. (2017).

[6] In the framework of PRO-RES project - PROmoting Ethics and Integrity in all Non-Medical RESearchtwo rounds of consultation were carried out, by thematic workshops, online interviews to 63 European experts and stakeholders. For more information, see Declich and Alfonsi (2020).

that (in the view of some interviewees) are likely to be increasingly challenged to go beyond the confines of academia and engage with society at large (Declich and Alfonsi 2020).

It must be noted, however, that despite their degree of scepticism about the usefulness of explicitly connecting research ethics with RRI, the research actors consulted showed awareness of the increasing demand on scientists and research institutions to be concerned with the social and political implications of their research.

So there can be a more substantive case for the contribution of RRI to the renewal of ethical discourse on science, based on the understanding that ethical issues are now strongly connected with the governance of science in the context of profound transformation. This entails managing continuous tensions between different levels of problems for institutions and individual scientists.

More importantly, as we will see in more detail in the next section, research ethics is challenged by the current evolution of science, which more and more requires a closer interaction between researchers and stakeholders, also reiterated by the EC presentation of the Horizon 2020 results (Monachello et al. 2020).

All in all, although RRI is not widely recognised and its use as an overarching label including research ethics is at least controversial, there seems to be a growing perception among research actors that the social status and role of science are changing, and radical transformations are affecting how science works and is organised, with important consequences for research ethics. This leads them to at least recognize that the issues and instances RRI is grounded on are real and, to some extent, shareable.

2.4 Analysis: A Policy Response to the Transformational Changes in Science and Society Relationships

In this section, based on the main elements presented in the previous paragraphs, some considerations will be proposed about the extent to which RRI may influence the discourse and practice of research ethics and integrity.

Quite paradoxically the potential relevance of RRI for research ethics should not be found in the inclusion of research ethics in the RRI conceptual structure as one of its structural components (the RRI keys). As discussed in the previous paragraphs, the simplistic incorporation of ethics in the RRI discourse might not be beneficial for strengthening research ethics, at least at a policy level. Rather, the connection between RRI and research ethics is deeper and more substantial: the same transformations affecting science that RRI intends to manage are inevitably also challenging the ethical dimension of research with equal force. In this sense, RRI starts being perceived not as a strategy to incorporate or replace research ethics, but as a support for ethically managing, from both a theoretical and methodological point of view, the multiple issues emerging from the rapid transformations of the research and innovation landscape.

The consulted literature, integrated with the results from the consultation, also allows the development of a first, although incomplete, picture of the challenges for research ethics arising from the transformations occurring in science and in science-society relationships. For the sake of simplicity, we can distinguish three types of challenges, respectively pertaining to major changes that are currently underway in the domains of research practices, research subjects, and research actors.

- Changes in research practices. Science is more and more globally interconnected, under continuous scrutiny and pressure by authorities and the public, hypercompetitive, and challenged by the shrinking of available funds and the growing demand for knowledge that is usable for policymaking and innovation.
- Changes in research subjects. ICTs and other emerging technologies combined with profound social transformations are giving birth to emerging phenomena leading to new socio-technical configurations. The emergence of radically new research fields, or the profound modification of existing ones, leads to new ethical implications.
- Change in the research actors. Finally, the types and number of players involved in the production of scientific knowledge are changing, with the growing involvement of non-scientific organisations. This is having an impact on research ethics (e.g., new conflicts of interest) or posing new issues susceptible to ethical consideration (e.g., the democratisation of the research process, responsibility for the research outputs, and the ethical soundness of research as a basis for evidence-based policies).

It is worth noticing that a growing awareness of the new ethical problems raised by the ongoing changes is emerging among researchers, research organisations, private companies, and policymakers, even if at different levels, depending on sectoral, geopolitical, and cultural differences. At the core of the ethical challenges, there seems to be an increasing uncertainty generated by the changes described above, which produces instability in the ways ethical issues emerge and are addressed. However, this process is at its very first stages. The analysis of the different sources used in this chapter suggests that research actors are well aware that the transformations occurring in science have a strong impact on the ethical sphere, but they are still far from developing a comprehensive view of the many issues involved.

Despite this, we have identified three priorities which are related to some of the four dimensions that appear as the more productive interpretation of the RRI approach (inclusiveness, anticipation, reflexivity, and responsiveness), respectively pertaining to the need to properly socially embed the research activity, to timely recognise and anticipate the implications of research, and to constantly find new and more appropriate ethical practices in research-related processes and outputs.

- **Contextualisation.** Effective research ethics needs to focus on research issues, which refer to different groups and interests. Science is more and more emerging as a societal enterprise which is increasingly called to orient evidence-based policies. This calls into question two dimensions of RRI, namely inclusiveness (asking for the involvement of all the concerned stakeholders) and reflexivity (claiming to constantly focus on the aims and results of ongoing activity so as not to lose their consistency).

- **Timely recognition and anticipation**. As emerged in the studies of new technologies, but not only limited to them, ethics is called to imagine uses and consequences of research and innovation for different social groups, as well as for society at large. This concept of ethics combines with three dimensions of RRI, i.e., anticipation (the need for anticipating the future implications, both positive and negative, of any new scientific output), inclusiveness, and responsiveness (calling on science to adopt strategies that detect risks early and develop ethically appropriate responses). Such dimensions are also very relevant for decision-makers and policymakers.
- **More effective ethical practices.** The third priority is that of constantly looking for more effective ethical ways to treat research-related processes and outputs. This means enlarging the scope of research ethics to encompass the entire research and innovation process, developing—when necessary—new methodologies and tools besides the traditional ones, on a case-by-case basis, and incorporating the practices adopted by all the relevant stakeholders, in a constant dialogue. This process of updating and innovating mainly relates to two RRI dimensions, i.e., reflexivity and responsiveness.

2.5 Lessons Learned

On the basis of the reasoning conducted in the previous paragraphs, we would like to draw some lessons from the rise of RRI in European policymaking up to Horizon 2020 and its apparent loss of centrality in the Horizon Europe Programme[7].

Of course—as we pointed out in the previous paragraphs—this experience has shown many drawbacks: the conceptual indetermination of the very concept, the risk of reification in turning RRI into just another label or a tick box exercise, and its limited currency among researchers and innovators. All this notwithstanding, some significant insights can be proposed.

The first lesson concerns the ability to mobilise resources—not only economic but also human and intellectual—that the RRI policy has produced in Europe, mainly through the Horizon 2020 programme (but also since the FP7 programme and through national initiatives, such as those of the United Kingdom Research and Innovation Council, or the Dutch Research Council), and outside Europe (e.g., in India, China, the USA, Brazil, etc.).[8] In this regard, RRI can be considered a powerful notion,

---

[7] In this we join other researchers that have been engaged in this field and are similarly reflecting about the RRI experience and making recommendations about its future (e.g., Owen et al. 2021; Stahl 2020; von Schomberg 2021).

[8] Numerous research organisations outside Europe have participated as partners in numerous FP7 and Horizon 2020 RRI projects. In addition, some countries have also launched RRI-inspired programmes (see Wittrock et al. 2021 and Owen et al. 2021).

thanks to its interpretive flexibility, its capacity to encompass other similar concepts (d'Andrea et al. 2017), and its capacity to mobilise actors of different types.

Secondly, the deployment of RRI policies produced a stock of knowledge and practices, including guidelines, roadmaps, and tools, able to capture the ongoing changes. As mentioned before, such stock of knowledge has been utilised to promote RRI-inspired institutional change[9] in universities and research organisations, as well as in local and regional public administrations, by activating societal actors, providing new frames and cultural inputs, and also, inevitably, meeting resistance and obstacles. Attempts to apply RRI have been tried out also in SMEs and industries,[10] especially in the fields of emerging technologies (ICTs, biotechnologies, etc.).

All these experiences contributed—and this is the third lesson—to the establishment of a community of practice, involving thousands of people that in recent years have been involved in studies, experiments, research projects and a myriad of reflexive initiatives (workshops, social labs, meetings, seminar, webinars, etc.).

The fourth lesson concerns the inspiration that the four dimensions of RRI can provide to the governance of science in the context of ongoing changes affecting both science itself and society. In this framework, RRI can be recognised as a regime of change, helping research institutions, researchers and other relevant actors to address changes affecting science (d'Andrea et al. 2017). Through this approach, attempts can be made to go beyond the logic of risk management in research towards a more comprehensive and effective governance of science.[11]

Furthermore, from the point of view of research ethics, these 10 years[12] have shown the need for a more dynamic, approach, to be able to navigate the uncertainty inherent in the contemporary research and innovation landscape, where new ethical dilemmas emerge as science and technology advance, and where a myriad of everyday big and small ethical problems emerge from research activities. Thus, the fifth lesson concerns research ethics as such. In this view, research ethics can no longer be developed only by scientists for scientists or prevalently based on deductive, top-down, and normative procedures. In this context, RRI (and in particular its four dimensions) could help to develop more proactive, flexible, anticipatory, inclusive, and exploratory ethical practices. This does not affect the entire picture of research ethics, but only part of it. In particular, it is possible to identify three main domains (Declich and Alfonsi 2020).

---

[9] See, for example, among others, the projects ACT, FIT4RRI, FOTRRIS, GRACE, JERRI, NUCLEUS, ORION, RESBIOS2, RRI PRACTICE; STAGES, SISCODE. Many projects were focused on gender equality.

[10] See for example, the projects Liv-In; ORBIT; New HoRRIzon; PRISMA; Responsible Industry; Responsible Innovation Compass; ROSIE; Smart Map.

[11] See for example, the projects DEEPEN, GREAT, FIT4RRI, RES-AGORA, SATORI.

[12] During these 10 years, several projects on ethics dealt with the complex issue to implement standards and provide regulatory framework for ethical research in field such as ICT, AI, robotics, HET, etc. and deepened the issues of ethics of emerging technologies, also making reference to RRI. See the projets ENERI, I-CONSENT, PANEFILT, PRO-RES, PRINTEGER, SIENNA, SHERPA, SOP4RI, TRUST, VIRT2UE.

The first domain includes the many research areas which are ethically stable, i.e., areas in which both ethical principles and ethical procedures are consolidated and still effective.

The second domain includes research areas which are more ethically unstable, i.e., areas in which the ethical principles are quite clear although the ethical procedures are partially or totally unclear. Think, for example, of areas such as research in public spaces, research in conflict and disaster areas, or internet-based research. In all these areas, the ethical principles are quite clear but the procedures for applying them are uncertain, since the traditional ones are increasingly ineffective.

The third domain includes research areas which are ethically new, i.e., areas for which neither the ethical principles nor the ethical procedures are clear. We are referring to cutting-edge research and technological domains, such as those related to AI, nanotechnologies, or human enhancement technologies, which are creating new social meanings, situations and configurations which need ethical interpretation.

Having identified these three areas, we can consider that often the research areas whose results are more acutely needed are those where the degree of uncertainty is higher. These areas are still under-socialised, i.e., they are not yet "filled", if perhaps partially, with those social meanings, contents, or experiences to make them socially manageable. The first to penetrate these areas are researchers and technicians, building their "social meanings" to interpret them. However, other players contribute to the socialisation process, including public authorities, experts, the different types of stakeholders involved and, eventually, ordinary citizens. It is in these frontier areas, where the relationships between science and society are more uncertain and problematic, that an approach to research that is proactive, anticipatory and inclusive can better ensure the quality of the results and their reliability for policymaking.

This consideration introduces the last lesson learned that, in our view, concerns the complex relationship between science and policymaking. Policymakers have been involved in RRI projects as stakeholders only to a small degree, but these 10 years have shown the need to deploy a system of mediation and hybridisation between policymakers and researchers with the involvement of dedicated figures. This implies that proper evidence-based policymaking should be seen as a transactional, multifaceted effort. In fact, even the best scientific evidence cannot be mechanically translated into policy. What is required is a complex, non-linear process that involves contextualisation, reflexivity, capacity to consult and interact with relevant actors and stakeholders, and anticipating risks and opportunities; in a word, the ability to consider those dimensions that are part and parcel of RRI.

2.6   Implications and Recommendations

On the basis of the path described so far, we would like to make some recommendations, based on the persuasion that even if RRI seems to be downplayed by the EU and losing its centrality in the governance of the relationship between science and society some elements of these 10 years should be, so to speak, "saved".

1. There is a need for a proactive, explorative and dynamic research ethics approach (or "ethics of future"[13]—EGE 2021) based on the practices and experimentation of the four dimensions of RRI in innovation and research activities. Such a proactive ethics approach can allow for more effective ethical management of the more unstable and newer research areas (the third and partially the second domain mentioned in the previous section).

2. As also suggested by others[14], there is a need for a scaling-up of the reflection on RRI (and its contents and challenges) from the level of individual research institutes to that of national and European research and innovation programmes. In this regard, there is the need to devise actual mechanisms for dialogue and co-creation involving researchers, stakeholders and policymakers.

3. Ethical reflexivity must be incorporated more into the mission-oriented innovation lines of Horizon Europe to help define their content and approaches. In this context, the space that RRI has provided over the past ten years, for debate, reflection, negotiation, and even dispute on the relationship between science, technology, responsibility and society, must be preserved, promoted and sustained (Owen et al. 2021).

4. The research centres, universities, industries, groups of researchers and stakeholders that have been mobilised over the years within the broad perspective of responsible research and innovation should be cared for, so that their valuable energy is not lost. There is a need to promote networking, synergies and platforms for the RRI communities of practice to continue their reflection and exchange of experiences (Owen et al. 2021). In this context, it is also appropriate to continue to experiment on how and under what conditions to promote institutional change in universities, research centres and industry for responsible, open and inclusive research and innovation.

5. There is a need for places and processes that allow researchers and policymakers to interact in order to address the socialisation of those areas of scientific and technological research that are progressing at a very fast pace so that their embeddedness in society is still weak, developed with scant interaction with the different stakeholders and with insufficient public control and assessment of their impacts, including considerable heterogeneity in the evaluation instruments. It is in this framework that evidence-based policymaking should be pursued as a transactional, multifaceted and interactive endeavour.

---

[13] In this regard, the European Group on Ethics in science and new technologies in its document "The role of ethics in European and global governance" underlies the need to a global engament of stakeholders, to use and practice ethics by design, to promote democratic deliberations and to involve ethics "in shaping the agenda".

[14] This is one of the element proposed during the New HoRRIzon Final Conference Session 7: H2020 to Horizon Europe: from ethical guidelines to democratic processes, held online on May 25, 2021.

References

Burget, M., E. Bardone, and M. Pedaste. 2017. Definitions and conceptual dimensions of responsible research and innovation: a literature review. *Science and Engineering Ethics*. 23: 1–19. https://doi.org/10.1007/s11948-016-9782-1.

Chadwick, R., and Z. Hub. 2013. Editorial: from ELSA to responsible research and promisomics. *Life Sciences, Society and Policy* 2013 (9): 3. https://doi.org/10.1186/2195-7819-9-3.

Charitidis, Costas, Eleni Spyrakou, Vassilis Markakis, and contribution by Ron Iphofen. 2019. Thematic priorities report. *Pro-RES Deliverable* D2: 1.

d'Andrea, Luciano, Marta Federico, Khama Nina and Vase Susanna. 2017. FIT4RRI D1.1–Report on the Literature Review. https://doi.org/10.5281/zenodo.1434349 https://zenodo.org/record/143 4349#.X8YFlM1Kg2x accessed 16 July 2021.

Declich, Giovanna, and Alfonso Alfonsi. 2020. Framework in the RRI context. *Pro-RES PROmoting Ethics and Integrity in Non-Medical RESearch–Deliverable* D3: 5.

Delaney, Niamh, Zeno Tornasi, Raluca Iagher, Roberta Monachello, and Colombe Warin. 2020. European Commission. Science with and for society in Horizon 2020. Achievements and Recommendations for Horizon Europe.

Eurobarometer. 2010. Science and technology report. Special Eurobarometer 340. Fieldwork: January 2010-February 2010. Publication: June 2010. European Commission.

Eurobarometer. 2013. Responsible research and innovation (RRI) Science and Technology. Report. Special Eurobarometer 401. European Commision.

European Commission. 2006. EURAB Activities Report 2005. European Communities.

European Commission. 2013. Options for strengthening responsible research and innovation. Report of the Expert Group on the State of Art in Europe on RRI. Publications Office of the European Union. https://doi.org/10.2777/46253.

European Commission. 2014. *Responsible research and innovation.* Europe's Ability to Respond to Societal Challenges: Publication Offices of the European Union.

European Group on Ethics in Science and New Technologies (EGE). 2021. Values for the future: the role of ethics in European and global governance. European Commission. https://ec.europa.eu/info/files/values-future-role-ethics-european-and-global-governance_en. Accessed 16 July 2021.

Geoghegan-Quinn, Máire. 2012. Message delivered at the Conference by Máire Geoghegan-Quinn, European Commissioner for Research, Innovation and Science. In *Science in dialogue. towards a european model for responsible research and innovation*, April 23–25, Odense, Denmark.

Grunwald, Armin. 2011. Responsible innovation: bringing together technology assessment, applied ethics, and STS research. *Enterprise and Work Innovation Studies* 7, IET:9–31.

Gumeirães Pereira, Angela, Tom Wakeford, Bruna De Marchi, Paula Curvelo, Sarah Davies, Inês Crespos, and Lucia Vesnic-Alejevic. 2013. Public engagement in scence and technology: setting the scene. JRC Working Paper. European Commission, Joint Research Centre.

House of Lords Select Committee on Science and Technology. 2000. Science and technology—third report. Session 1999–2000. https://publications.parliament.uk/pa/ld199900/ldselect/ldsctech/38/3801.htm. Accessed 20 Aug 2021.

Kalichman, M. 2013. A brief history of RCR education. *Research* 20 (5–6): 380–394. https://doi.org/10.1080/08989621.2013.822260.

Lubberink, R., V. Blok, J. van Ophem, and O. Omta. 2017. Lessons for responsible innovation in the business context: a systematic titerature review of responsible, social and sustainable innovation practices. *Sustainability.* 9 (721): 1–31. https://doi.org/10.3390/su9050721.

Monachello, R., Z. Tornasi, and N. Delaney. 2020. Research ethics and research integrity: Achievements in Horizon 2020 and recommendations on the way forward. https://doi.org/10.2777/63976.

Owen, R., P. Macnaghten, and J. Stilgoe. 2012. Responsible research and innovation: from science in society to science for society, with society. *Science and Public Policy.* 39: 751–760. https://doi.org/10.1093/scipol/scs093.

Owen, Richard, and Mario Pansera. 2019. Responsible innovation and responsible research and innovation. In *Handook on science and public policy*, eds. Simon Dagmar, Kuhlmann Stefan, Stamm Julia and Canzler Weert. Edward Elgar publishing.

Owen, Richard, Jack Stilgoe, Phil Macnaghten, Mike Gorman, Erik Fisher, and Dave H. Guston. 2013. Framework for responsible innovation. In *Responsible Innovation*, 1st Edn, eds. Owen, Richard, Heintz, Maggy and Bessant, John R. John Wiley & Sons, Ltd.

Owen, R., J. Stilgoe, P. Macnaghten, M. Gorman, E. Fisher, and D. H. Guston. 2018. Methods for practising ethics in research and innovation: a literature review, critical analysis and recommendations. *Science and Engineering ethics*. https://doi.org/10.1007/s11948-017-9961-8.

Owen, Richard, René von Schomberg, and Phil Macnaghten. 2021. An unfinished journey? Reflections on a decade of Responsible Research and Innovation. *Journal of Responsible Innovation* 8(2): 217–233. https://doi.org/10.1080/23299460.2021.1948789

Rip, Arie. 2016. Responsible Research and Innovation (RRI). The many lives of responsible research and innovation. *Euroscientist. European science conversations by the community, for the community*. Special Issue. https://www.euroscientist.com/rri-fashion/. Accessed 4 July 2021.

Stahl, B.C. 2013. Responsible research and innovation: the role of privacy in an emerging framework. *Science and Public Policy* 40: 708–716. https://doi.org/10.1093/scipol/sct067.

Stahl, B. C. 2020. Emerging technologies as the next pandemic? Possible consequences of the Covid crises for the future of the future of responsible research and innovation. *Ethics and Information technology* https://doi.org/10.1007/s10676-020-09551-1.

Stilgoe, O. R., and P. Macnaghten. 2013. Developing a framework for responsible innovation. *Research Policy* 42:1568–1580. https://doi.org/10.1016/j.respol.2013.05.008.

Timmermans, Job, and Bernd Carsten Stahl. 2013. Annual Report on the main trends of SiS, in particular, the trends related to RRI. GREAT Governance of Responsible Innovation. Deliverable D6.4. https://www.great-project.eu/deliverables_files/deliverables05. Accessed 16 July 2021.

van den Hoven, Jeroen. 2014. Responsible innovation in brief. The Delft University of Technology. https://d1rkab7tlqy5f1.cloudfront.net/TBM/Over%20faculteit/Afdelingen/Values%2C%20Technology%20and%20Innovation/People/Full%20Professors/Responsible_Innovation_in_brief.pdf. Accessed 30 June 2021.

von Schomberg, René. 2011. Introduction. Towards responsible research and innovation in the information and communication technologies and security technologies fields. In *Towards responsible research and innovation in the information and communication technologies and security technologies fields*. von Schomberg, René. (Ed.). European Commission.

von Schomberg, R. 2012. Prospects for technology assessment in a framework of responsible research and innovation. In *Technikfolgen abschätzen lehren. VS Verlag für Sozialwissenschaften*, eds. Dusseldorp Marc and Beecroft Richard, 39–61. https://doi.org/10.1007/978-3-531-934 68-6_2.

von Schomberg, René. 2019. Why responsible innovation. In *The International handbook on responsible innovation. A global resource*, eds. von Schomberg, René and Jonathan Hankins, 12–32. Edward Elgar Publishing.

von Schomberg, R. 2021. Interview. Dr. René von Schomberg, directorate general for research and innovation of the European Commission, discusses responsible innovation, open science, and game changers. *OMICS A Journal of Integrative biology* 25(6):333–335. https://doi.org/10.1089/omi.2021.0066.

Wellcome Global Monitor. 2018. How does the world feel about science and health. Gallup. Wellcome Trust. https://wellcome.org/sites/default/files/wellcome-global-monitor-2018.pdf. Accessed 20 Aug 2021.

Wittrock, Christian, Auke Pols, David Ludwig, Ellen-Marie Forsberg, and Philip Macnaghten. 2021. *Implementing Responsible Research and Innovation*. Cham: Springer.

Wynne, Brian and Ulrike Felt. 2007. European Commission. Taking European knowledge society seriously. Report of the Expert Group on Science Governance to the Science, economy and Society Directorate, Directorate-General for Research, European Commission.

Chapter 3
Responsible Research and Innovation and India: A Case for Contextualization and Mutual Learning

Krishna Ravi Srinivas

Abstract Responsible Research and Innovation (RRI) is largely identified as a concept developed in Europe and adopted mostly in Europe, particularly in research. Principles in RRI have been incorporated into policies and programs in Europe and elsewhere. While studies have pointed out the need to adapt/contextualize/transduce RRI in non-European countries and contexts, the extent to which this is possible is a big issue. Developing countries like China are adopting and contextualizing RRI to suit their needs and to enhance protocols/practices. this chapter takes India as an example and points out that RRI is relevant for India and at the same time some of the keys in RRI find a place in Science, Technology, and Innovation (STI) policy and practice, although RRI as a concept is not acknowledged or recognized. This chapter argues that contextualizing RRI for India, particularly in the light of STI Policy (STIP) (under finalization) and Scientific Social Responsibility (SSR) is feasible and desirable. While the former gives importance to Open Science, Science Education (in the Indian context), Science Communication and Gender, SSR opens up possibilities for enriching RRI. Similarly, RRI in theory and practice can benefit from interaction with ideas and practices developed in India such as Access, Equity and Inclusion, Scientific Temper and Scientific Social Responsibility. These ideas and practices may not be relevant in all countries in adopting RRI but can contribute to the diversity in RRI as a concept and practice.

Keywords Responsible research and innovation · Science-society · Science · Technology and innovation · Contextualization · Access · Equity and inclusion · India

K. R. Srinivas (✉)
Research and Information System for Developing Countries (RIS), India Habitat Center, Lodi Road,
New Delhi, India
e-mail: ravisrinivas@ris.org.in

© The Author(s) 2022
D. O'Mathúna and R. Iphofen (eds.), *Ethics, Integrity and Policymaking*, Research Ethics Forum 9, https://doi.org/10.1007/978-3-031-15746-2_3

3.1 Introduction

RRI has emerged as an important concept and practice in Science, Technology and Innovation (STI). The origin of RRI can be traced to the Sixth Framework Program (FP6) Program of the European Commission which was from 2002–2006 and established a new program 'Science and Society' with one of the objectives of the Program being to encourage 'responsible research and application of science and technology' (Owen et al. 2021). This emphasis on 'responsible research and application' received further thrust in the Seventh Framework Program (FP7) and the subsequent program Horizon 2020. Over the past decade or so, the idea of RRI received much traction within Europe and elsewhere.

A working definition of RRI is: "Responsible research and innovation is an approach that anticipates and assesses potential implications and societal expectations with regard to research and innovation, with the aim to foster the design of inclusive and sustainable research and innovation" (European Commission 2020). Another much cited definition is: "Responsible Research and Innovation is a transparent, interactive process by which societal actors and innovators become mutually responsive to each other with a view on the (ethical) acceptability, sustainability and societal desirability of the innovation process and its marketable products (in order to allow a proper embedding of scientific and technological advances in our society)" (Von Schomberg 2011, 9). In 2012, the then EU Commissioner for Research, Innovation and Science Máire Geoghegan-Quinn affirmed high-level EC policy support for RRI by stating "our duty as policy makers [is] to shape a governance framework that encourages responsible research and innovation" (Geoghegan-Quinn 2012).

The objective of this approach is to align the process and outcome of the innovation process with the needs, expectations, and values of the society. This calls for stakeholders, ranging from scientists and researchers to users/consumers, working together to achieve this with a shared understanding. The idea of RRI keys is used to elucidate this. In RRI the six keys or dimensions are public engagement, gender equality, science education, open access, ethics, and governance (European Commission 2004). Anticipation and Reflection are key components of RRI. According to the ORBIT Project, "The key to anticipation for RRI is to ensure that consequences of undertaking the research and of possible findings are considered and that these considerations are reflected in the research design… One way of describing reflection in RRI is to see it as an example of second order reflexivity, i.e., of a reflection on the processes of reflection that underpin and guide research. This means that the axioms and basic assumptions need to be questioned with a view to ensuring that the research is aligned with societal needs and requirements" (ORBIT no date).

Smith et al. (2019) point out that Owen, Stilgoe, Macnaghten and the Engineering and Physical Sciences Research Council (EPSRC) of the United Kingdom developed the Anticipation, Inclusion, Reflexivity, Responsiveness (AIRR) framework. This framework and the Anticipation and Reflection mentioned by the European Commission are similar, but not identical. Anticipate means consider the future path of research or research and development and think in terms of potential plausible consequences and impacts. Seeking voices and views of a broad range of stakeholders is Inclusion, while reflections on the paths and directions chosen and considered is Reflexivity. Responsiveness means including and integrating the outcomes of the first three processes (Anticipate, Inclusion and Reflexivity). The AIRR framework is more expansive than Anticipation and Reflection, but it also depends on how the terms are interpreted and applied. Moreover, the differences in translating these into praxis cannot be ignored. As EPSRC has co-developed the AIRR framework, it is used more in the projects related to RRI funded by EPSRC whereas projects on RRI funded by the European Commission use Anticipation and Reflection more than the AIRR framework.

RRI has been the theme of many research projects and the literature has increased significantly. For example, using Web of Science, Ortt et al. (2020), found that the number of articles published on responsible innovation increased from less than 10 in 1994 to about 500 in 2018. The RRI framework or the concept of RRI and its relevance has been studied and discussed in different contexts, along with its application in governance of STI, particularly in emerging technologies such as nanotechnology, synthetic biology, Information and Communication Technologies (ICT) and neurotechnologies.

Although RRI and Responsible Innovation (RI) have been used interchangeably in the literature they are not the same. While RRI is a broad concept and practice that involves both research and innovation and gives emphasis to science education, RI has a distinct focus on innovation. RI does not have Science Education as a dimension. Tracing the roots of RI to the Dutch Research Council's Program on Socially Responsible Innovations, Jeroen van den Hoven (2017, 2) points out that, "Responsible innovation can, as a concept, be understood in a substantive and in a procedural sense. As a procedural notion, responsible innovation refers to a process of innovation that meets certain procedural norms, like accountability, inclusiveness, due care and transparency (to stakeholders and to society). As a substantive notion, responsible innovation refers to results and outcomes of innovation processes in the form of products, systems or services, i.e., innovative technologies, which reflect and accommodate moral values."

In contrast, RRI takes a broader perspective on research, innovation and society and the governance framework and dimensions go beyond what is envisaged in RI. Although there are similarities and a strong emphasis on connection with society and stakeholders in both, RRI is much broader and has wider connotations in terms of concept, discourse and practice. In that sense, RRI is more relevant for STI (Science, Technology and Innovation) policy making than RI. RI is more appropriate for innovation-related planning and development activities, particularly in the industrial sector.

Irrespective of the term used, RRI and RI have added a new dimension to theory and practice in understanding and working in science-society relationship. This does not necessarily mean that they have replaced approaches and practices like Technology Assessment, Ethical, Legal and Social Impact (ELSI) Assessment or the typical cost–benefit analysis (CBA). But there are questions about the relevance of

RRI and RI, their adoption in different sectors and whether they can be adopted beyond Europe, particularly in the Global South.

In this regard, this chapter's objective is modest: to discuss the contextualization of RRI in India and what RRI as a concept and practice can learn from India. My contention is that RRI is relevant for India but must be contextualized and that contextualization has to be sensitive to issues in STI in India and the societal needs in India. RRI can learn and adopt some aspects from policies and practices in India and an RRI contextualized for India will be a hybrid that takes the best from RRI concept and practice from India and elsewhere. The recent (draft) Science, Technology and Innovation Policy (STIP), which is yet to be officially approved, creates many opportunities for this although the Policy does not use the concept of RRI or RI (Department of Science and Technology DST 2020). STIP is an outcome of an exercise undertaken jointly by the Department of Science and Technology (DST) and the Office of Principal Scientific Advisor. It is a successor to the 2013 STI Policy. It is expected to give a major boost to STI in India and enable India to meet inter alia, self-sufficiency ('Atma Nirbhar') in many sectors including in strategic sectors. As the policy is not official, I am using the draft of the policy which was put up for public comment as the reference (Department of Science and Technology DST 2020).

3.2 Responsible Research and Innovation

3.2.1 RRI in Europe

Many of the research projects on RRI have addressed its application in different sectors, issues in measuring and developing indicators, comparative analysis of interpretation, and application of RRI in different countries. RRI has been integrated into policy documents or policy processes in some countries. In some, the core ideas of RRI have been acknowledged or adopted in policymaking. On the other hand, there are criticisms and self-reflexive accounts of RRI, interestingly mostly from those who are associated with projects on RRI. Coenen (2016) opined that conceptual work in RRI may be deemed as a process innovation and underscores the need to broaden the discourse on RRI.

As Fisher (2020) points out, there are positive developments regarding RRI as it gains support from policy makers and funders, and RRI per se or concepts from it are integrated into new programs in Science, Technology and Innovation. Still, as he points out, there is a need to rethink how it is conceptualized, introduced and implemented. After reflecting upon a decade of RRI and comparing it to a conversation, Owen, Schomberg and Macnaghten state, "It has played its part in helping us to understand, reflect on and open up those futures being created by science, technology and innovation, and how we can take responsibility for those futures as a society" (2021, 13). But taking a critical perspective Novitzky et al. (2020) point out that while the EU promoted RRI in principle, its implementation was problematic.

Although RRI as a concept has been developed in Europe and supported by the EC and some funding agencies, the adoption of RRI has been limited. Christensen et al. (2020) point out that there are many issues with RRI in theory as well as in implementation, ranging from weakness in concept, lack of indicators and tools for assessment, to justifying RRI's relevance and importance vis a vis former practices. Of course, the seven hindrances they cite, such as lack of funding or lack of political support, would be true in most circumstances or countries. They point out that as there are many initiatives to promote RRI practices, the concept itself may be of less importance. This results in a dilemma. Should this be taken as a positive acknowledgment of RRI and absorbing its principles through practice although not in the name of RRI or does it mean that while RRI practices have more practical relevance while theory per se has less use or relevance?

It is possible to use the emphasis on RRI keys in RRI without indicating that RRI is their source of inspiration. Certainly, while some initiatives would have incorporated some of the keys, without labelling their origin in RRI, due incorporation of the others would enhance the responsibility dimension without any reference to RRI. According to Novitzky et al., "The lack of clarity in conceptualizing RRI for research policy and governance, the limited understanding among key stakeholders, and the concept's conflation with other—often conflicting—policy goals (e.g., scientific excellence, economic value, technological readiness) hinder the emergence of a specific RRI-oriented policy frame" (2020, 41).

The other case studies from the RRI Practice and Nucleus projects also show the divergences in understanding and implementation of RRI within Europe and outside Europe. For example, Owen et al. (2019) state that most institutions understand and implement 'ethics' as a matter of research ethics and scientific integrity while only some give serious attention to reflecting on impacts on society. In this and related matters there is no consistency or uniformity even among institutions in Europe. But the impact of projects on RRI has been significant and a review by the European Commission (European Commission 2020a) points out that about 250 individual institutional change plans are implemented or being implemented and in about 130 institutions Gender Equality Plans (GEPs) have been implemented or are under implementation.

Thus, it can be safely concluded that despite criticisms, RRI has become an important concept and practice in STI at least in Europe. The continuing support by the European Commission and funding agencies, research projects that are expanding the application of RRI, and active interest from academics and stakeholders are ensuring that RRI is getting more firmly embedded in the theory and practice of innovation in Europe.

3.2.2 RRI Beyond Europe

Many aspects of RRI have been questioned, including the idea of 'Responsible' and its conceptual basis. For example, Valkenburg et al. (2020) bring in issues of exclusion and the need to empower diverse epistemologies. They suggest this based on a single case study, and for a problem that is confined to a few states in India and to a problem that itself is seasonal. I cite this as an example to argue that RRI as a concept and practice has attracted much attention as well as criticism. In later sections, I will provide suggestions to make it more relevant and meaningful, and seek to expand its scope and diversify its ambit.

But what is the right approach to make RRI more relevant and meaningful across various countries, cultures and systems of innovation? According to Doezema et al. (2019), transduction is a better approach as that would make RRI a truly global concept that does not seek to standardize and creates space for multiple knowledges without instrumentalization. Thus, transduction could mean development of novel concepts related to RRI and deeper and better engagement with RRI which can be context-specific. For example, resource constraint may not be an issue for a funding body in Europe which emphasizes RRI in assessing projects, while in a developing country resource constraint can be an issue and a funding body may promote development of innovations that are effective and cheaper as an example of responsible innovation or consider that aspect in a project as a positive factor representing a dimension of RRI in that context. There are case studies on development of cheaper, in-house built instruments and research equipment in the global South.

Asveld and Dam-Mieras (2018) argue that there is a need to accept alternative conceptual structures and contextualize RRI. Jakobsen et al. (2019) take a position that it is also important to broaden the concept of innovation under RRI and it should go beyond what is done in laboratories or by scientists. Recent literature on RRI (e.g., Ortt et al. 2020) includes case studies on large technological systems and frugal innovation. This indicates that RRI in discourse and practice is moving beyond innovations that emanate from typical Research and Development (R&D) processes to include diversity in innovations. Typical R&D processes are done in academic or research institutions or in industry so that from basic research, innovations are developed.

RRI's relevance and utility in non-European contexts has also attracted much attention, mostly from national case studies and comparative analyses made in different research projects in RRI such as RRI Practice (https://rri-practice.eu). But was RRI conceptualized primarily with European society and its values in mind or to address the Science-Society-Innovation issues in Europe? In a much-cited paper on RRI, Stilgoe et al. state "in different cultural contexts, different values will be more or less pertinent, and they may be conflicted. In our analysis, we have therefore been reticent to explicitly define the normative ends of responsible innovation" (2013, 1577).

Irrespective of this reticence, over the years the major question has been about how relevant RRI is for non-European countries and in non-European contexts. In the last three or four years, studies have been published on RRI done in large countries like

Brazil and China on how it has been adopted and perceived there. The literature points to multiple versions and pathways related to responsible innovation. For example, according to Yan and Ravesteijn, "This Chinese context, in which this development takes place, differs from conditions in Europe and the United States. In addition, China, the EU and America are confronted with similar but not completely overlapping environmental and social challenges. All of this results in different pathways and versions of responsible innovation" (2019, 117).

This raises an important question: is the concept of RRI a sort of procrustean bed to define and measure innovation? Other questions arise about how to assess innovations that are often bottom-up solutions that are developed more as workable and affordable innovations that meet societal needs using the keys of RRI and the RRI principles. This is an issue not just for frugal innovation but also for inclusive innovation and grassroots innovation.

Vasen (2017) has pointed out that RI should not be restricted to emerging technologies and should be sensitive to developments and needs of and in developing countries, and calls for a dialog between RI and inclusive innovation so that an integrated framework can be developed. Although RRI and RI are different, both are relevant for developing socially responsible innovations in emerging technologies in different national contexts.

On similar lines, Bhaduri and Talat (2020) suggest that there should be a dialog between frugal innovation and RRI. Hartley et al. (2019) suggest that some elements of RI can be transferable to the South and, referring to the view of Biddle, they suggest that a technology that addresses a locally defined societal need, with research done in the local context and results accessible to those who need it most, can be considered as RI.

Thus, it can be stated that a consensus exists among academics working on RRI/RI, that there is a need to go beyond the conventional approaches and conceptualizations of RRI/RI as well as to critically engage with new ideas, concepts, and practices. This is a welcome development. Even as such a consensus emerges, we have case studies on RRI/RI in developing countries, particularly from the RRI Practice Project (https://rri-practice.eu) and Nucleus Project (https://www.nucleus-project.eu/). The case studies reveal that the response to RRI has been mixed. For example, the case study from Brazil points out many hurdles for RRI in Brazil. The report from India points out that RRI is perceived as a novel concept and is virtually unknown in India although there is interest among academics and policy makers to know more about it.

In China, while there have been positive developments in terms of RRI getting recognized among policy makers and in policy documents, besides being adopted in large infrastructure projects, there are constraints too. According to Gao et al., "As we have shown, entry points for RRI can be identified across broad domains of Chinese society, where quite a number of promising practices are emerging. However, there lacks an institutional mechanism for dialogue and for exchanges to take place across different levels" (2019, 372).

The 13th Five-Year National Science and Technology Innovation Program (2016) in China advocates, inter alia, RRI. But the interpretation of RRI is different from that of the European Commission. According to Mei et al., "Thus, RI is framed differently in the EU and China. The EU adopts a more political perspective, meaning that RI is mainly framed in terms of inclusiveness and open access, and implemented through a systemic policy program. In contrast, China, a highly centralized and emerging country, appears to be more ethically oriented, namely, it mostly focuses on the individual responsibilities of scientists and firms rather than claiming profound transformations at governance level" (2020, 1).

This divergence is inevitable given the differences in political structures and values that underpin the Science, Technology and Innovation ecosystem or the National Innovation System. Still, that does not mean that there is no possibility for mutual learning or having similar views on issues like ethical governance in certain technologies and applications (e.g., human germline modification, human genome editing) where RRI can play a key role in governance as it has ethics and public engagement as keys and strives to inculcate anticipation and reflexivity among scientists and institutions. Since there is a reference to RRI in official documents in China, which seem to advocate RRI, this could be considered as a case of transduction or contextualization. I am not sure, but I think this is more a case of contextualization than transduction. According to a report from Nucleus Project (2017), in China and South Africa, elements of RRI were conceptualized via various and different notions and there were some common features at the level of policies, such as giving emphasis to science education, or giving importance to innovation and knowledge economy. Similarly, Setiawan, (2018) pointed out the need to consider cultural aspects explicitly for RRI to become more relevant in different contexts.

Wakunuma et al. (2021) point out that hybrid forms of RRI can emerge and they cite Brazil as an example. After a comparative analysis of RRI in The Netherlands, Brazil and Malawi they conclude: "Mutual learning across regional and sector boundaries appears to be key to an open, fluid, internationally inclusive RRI approach that can be adapted to global contexts and towards an integrated conceptual framework of RRI moving forward into the future" (2021, 19).

The above discussion on understanding and applying RRI/RI makes it obvious that wide variance exists, and this has resulted in calls for expanding definitions of RRI or taking country-specific aspects into consideration in deploying RRI, whether it is in the North or South.

3.3 RRI and India

3.3.1 RRI and Its Relevance for India

The debates on the role of science in society preceded India's independence in 1947 and since them the thrust has been towards the application of science for the benefit of society (Chaturvedi and Srinivas, 2015). The S&T Vision 2032 Document of the NITI Aayog, an apex premier policy 'think tank' of the Government of India, has emphasized using S&T for addressing various societal challenges such as safe drinking water, affordable healthcare, food security, clean air, etc. (NITI Aayog 2017). India adopted the Green Revolution to increase output in agriculture and the White Revolution to make the country self-sufficient in the dairy sector (Pingali 2012, Scholten 2010).

A key objective of founding the Indian Space Research Organization (ISRO), which has gained a reputation for developing and launching low-cost high-capability satellites, was the application of space technology for societal benefit. Nanotechnology has been supported through Nano-Mission, a multi-year programme (Beumer 2019). Nano-Mission has funded projects that resulted in affordable innovations in water purification and supply. Thus, meeting societal needs and aspirations has been a key feature of India's endeavours in S&T. These and most of the innovation-related initiatives and projects in India emanate from a top-down approach while India is also known for its grassroots innovations and frugal innovations (Abraham 2021a, b).

The concept of RRI is not part of the official discourse on S&T, although many elements of RRI, including gender and science education, are present in various policies and programs in different forms (Srinivas et al. 2018). Over the years, the Department of Science and Technology (DST) has promoted initiatives to enhance participation of women in S&T. In recent years, open access and open data have been given importance. DST is supporting science communication through an organization called Vigyan Parsar. These have nothing to do with the concept of RRI even though promoting some of the keys (public engagement, open access, gender, science education) has become part of the policy. Most of them preceded the concept of RRI and are implemented for specific objectives. For example, the DST has six different programs, including the Indo-US Fellowship for Women in STEMM, to empower women and promote gender equality in science. Elsewhere I have pointed out that the ideas and initiatives of Kumarappa and Reddy can be considered as pioneering ones in RRI in India although they did not use that term (Srinivas and Pandey 2019).

India has been adopting international guidelines in ethics, including those pertaining to research involving human subjects. Recently the revised Guidelines on Ethics has been adopted by the Indian Council on Medical Research (ICMR 2017) and the Guidelines discuss Responsible Research. Institutional ethics committees and mandatory clearances are part of the research/project review and funding process. With respect to clinical trials, international standards and the need to adhere to global norms to get legitimacy and acceptability were factors for changes in law and practice.

Although public engagement is not part of the official S&T policy, the 2018 Economic Survey stressed the importance of public engagement and communication (Ministry of Finance, 2017). Civil society institutions have been doing science communication and public engagement. The journal of the Indian Science Academy (ISA), entitled *Dialog*, is focused on science communication and engagement with the wider public. Although the RRI keys are important for India, RRI cannot be transplanted into India using the same discourse and ideas on ethics, public engagement and reflexivity. Contextualization and examining their relevance for India is necessary as otherwise RRI will remain an alien concept with little relevance.

For example, open science in the Indian context also means access to textbooks and course materials, particularly in regional languages, and not just access to scientific literature in journals and data. Similarly, gender and science in the Indian context cannot be divorced from the historical under-representation of women in science and the various factors and barriers in Indian society (some of which, like caste inequalities, are specific to India) that constrain fuller and better participation of women in science, or for that matter in higher education and research.

Contextualizing the concept and practice of RRI for India is a challenge, but not an impossible one. As India continues to invest heavily in S&T and aspires to be in the top league among countries in S&T, understanding and applying RRI in India will help in developing innovations needed by society, and based on ethics and public engagement. This may result in better acceptance and maybe avoid unnecessary controversies over innovations. There are new and upcoming initiatives, including missions and national plans, in Artificial Intelligence, Cognitive Science and Internet of Things (IoT). In all three domains, the literature on RRI is growing and India can learn lessons from this which will complement contextualization of RRI in India.

3.3.2 Science, Technology and Innovation Policy (STIP) (Draft) and RRI

In 2020 DST and the Office of Principal Scientific Advisor (oPSA) launched an initiative to prepare a new Science, Technology and Innovation Policy (STIP). The previous STI policy elicited mixed responses and there were critiques (e.g., Krishna 2013). While adopted in 2013, it was not followed up with a strategy to implement it. Since 1947, there have been four policy statements, Scientific Policy Resolution of 1958 (Government of India 1958), Technology Policy Statement 1983 (Department of Science and Technology DST 1983), Science and Technology Policy of 2003 (Department of Science and Technology DST 2003) and Science, Technology and Innovation Policy (Department of Science and Technology DST 2013). Abraham (2021a, b) has analyzed these.

When the National Democratic Alliance (NDA) was elected to power in 2014, the then Planning Commission was dissolved and a new entity, NITI Aayog, was established. Previously, India had adopted five-year plans after becoming independent in 1947 which were modelled after the Soviet Union's experience with five-year planning. The distinct feature of these five-year plans was that they had a specific chapter on science which outlined the priorities and goals of the country in Science and Technology (S&T). In addition to the strategies outlined in these plans, special programs and missions were initiated to meet specific objectives. Until 1991, the thinking was based on state-led planning that emphasised a strong public sector, giving priority to S&T for societal needs and objectives under the five-year plans.

The state decided the direction and purpose of S&T in India and invested heavily in public sector institutions in S&T as well as in public sector units in different sectors.

This largely command-and-control approach underwent a change in 1991 when the economy opened up through liberalization, globalization and policy changes that enlarged the space and freedom for the private sector in almost all sectors. Still the government did not give up five-year plans, nor the idea that the state should play a major role in S&T, although private sector R&D was encouraged and incentivized. The last Five-Year Plan was for 2012–2017 but as the new government took over in 2014 and dissolved the Planning Commission, the idea of five-year plans was abandoned. However, the structure and organisation of S&T in government did not change. Thus, there is continuity and change in S&T in government. In terms of Gross Expenditure on R&D, about 65% is from the public sector while the rest is from private sector. Since 2014 there has been a greater thrust on digitization and using digitization and Information and Communication Technologies (ICT) for effective delivery of public services and to enhance financial inclusion and food security.

STIP (Department of Science and Technology DST 2020), while not explicitly mentioning RRI or discussing responsible innovation as a guiding concept, has many ideas, proposals and initiatives that are directly related to RRI and its keys. For example, it gives a strong emphasis to open access and open science, outlining the need to expand and enhance access to scientific knowledge, data and infrastructure. It has a Chapter on Equity and Inclusion focused on enhancing the role and contribution of women in science. It has conceptualized Gender in a broader way and considers exclusion on account of other factors and categories of exclusion. It has proposed adaptation of the Athena-SWAN model for transforming institutions and for promoting equity and inclusion in them. The importance to science education is clearly mentioned in the chapter on Capacity Building and in other places in the document. Science Communication and public engagement are discussed in a separate chapter with more emphasis on science communication, although the importance of public engagement is recognized in a limited manner.

Mr. Narendra Modi, the Prime Minister of India, in his address to the annual Indian Science Congress in 2019, mentioned the Social Responsibility of scientists. This has resulted in DST developing a concept of Scientific Social Responsibility (SSR). The draft STIP states the following regarding SSR: "2.1.6 Students of all educational levels will be given opportunities to get exposure to be part of leading science laboratories during the period of end-term breaks as part of Scientific Social Responsibility Policy" (Department of Science and Technology DST 2020, 17). In addition: "8.3.1 In line with the national policy on Scientific Social Responsibility (SSR 2020), and, scientists and researchers will be motivated and incentivised to engage in Science Communication and Public Engagement Activities. Institutes and organizations will be encouraged to earmark a percentage of allocated budget (SSR fund) for science communication and public engagement activities" (Department of Science and Technology DST 2020, 46).

Based on the SSR policy draft of 2019, and the concepts of SSR and RRI, Braun et al. (2020) have made some suggestions for DST and EC to work together and further mutual learning in RRI and enrich both SSR and RRI in theory and practice. In May 2022, DST published *Scientific Social Responsibility (SSR) Guidelines*. SSR is defined as "The ethical obligation of knowledge workers in all fields of science and technology to voluntarily contribute their knowledge and resources to the widest spectrum of stakeholders in society, in a spirit of service and conscious reciprocity" (Department of Science and Technology DST 2022, 12).

These guidelines can be useful for strengthening science-society linkages and encourage scientists and technocrats to spend more time and energy in science communication and reach out to educational institutions and students, and to the neighbourhoods in which they operate. These official Guidelines provide much scope for creative engagement by scientists and scientific institutions. The activities envisaged are varied and institutions have flexibility in using them. On the other hand, these are based (although not stated) on a 'deficit in public understanding model'. In this it is the public that needs to be made aware of, communicated about and educated. Many of the proposed activities are based on this assumption. Although it is stated, "Society-science connect: Collaborating with communities to identify their needs and problems and develop scientific and technological solutions. The age-old approach of Lab to Land (L2) would be replaced by a new-age approach of Land (Experience) to Lab (Expertise) to Land (Applications) (L3)" (Department of Science and Technology DST 2022, 4). But SSR Guidelines do not give scope for learning from communities and learning with communities. Nor do they envisage engaging with citizen science, Do-It-Yourself Biology or Makers and Hackers. The guidelines envisage that support from SSR-related activities will be from multiple sources and funds through Corporate Social Responsibility mechanisms. Thus, institutions need not rely solely on funds from the government to implement SSR.

As the guidelines have just been issued, it is too early to know about their implementation. SSR guidelines indicate the desire to give effect to the concept of SSR and make it part of science-related activities undertaken by institutions. It would have been better had the SSR guidelines taken into account recent developments in theory and practice in Public Understanding of Science and Public Engagement in Science. Nonetheless SSR guidelines will enable more active engagement by scientific institutions with society. From a RRI perspective this is a welcome development.

Although there has not been a distinct Indian version of RRI, I am of the view that based on India's experiences with S&T and concepts and practices developed in India, India can enrich and contribute to RRI in theory and practice. To illustrate this, I provide two examples.

3.3.3 Scientific Temper

The Constitution of India may be the only one that specifies cultivation of scientific temper as a fundamental duty. According to Article 51 of the Constitution of India "it shall be the duty of every citizen of India to develop the scientific temper, humanism and the spirit of inquiry and reform." This duty is not mandatory and is only a suggestion. Scientific temper and spirit of inquiry reflect the Enlightenment values that are at the core of modern humanism. The Constitution also indicates that the spirit of inquiry is part of the fundamental duty. Spirit of inquiry can inform public engagement and can justify it. In my view the concept of scientific temper can be developed further in the context of Science, Technology and Innovation and may be used in discourse and practice in RRI. Scientific temper is not a methodology but an attitude and an approach to understanding and action (Mahanti 2013).

Jawahar Lal Nehru, the first Prime Minister of India, articulated the idea of scientific temper in his book *The Discovery of India* (Nehru 1946). Since then, it has been discussed and debated in India and elsewhere. Nehru articulated Scientific Temper not as an attitude that worships science but as an attitude that has scope for self-reflection and critical inquiry. Although I will not elaborate on this point further, the idea of scientific temper has scope to be examined in the light of debates over RRI and understanding of science education and communication, and public engagement, particularly in developing countries. In these days of disinformation, fake news, climate change denial, and anti-vaccine campaigns, it is relevant in the North as well. In terms of RRI keys, Scientific Temper is closely related to ethics, science education, citizen engagement and governance while the elements of reflexivity and anticipation are included also. It is suggested that its relevance for RRI and RI can be explored, and the concept of Scientific Temper can be adopted and contextualized.

3.3.4 Access, Equity and Inclusion and RRI

Chaturvedi and Srinivas (2015) have identified Access, Equity and Inclusion (AEI) as values that can be used to assess the outcomes of S&T and Innovation policies in developing countries. This approach is compatible with inclusive development and can also be related to inclusive innovation. As a preliminary exercise we highlight how Access, Equity and Inclusion can be compared with the keys in RRI and also with some of the policies proposed in STIP (Department of Science and Technology DST 2020). The following table attempts to provide an overview of Indian keys of AEI in relation to RRI and STIP. STIP does not use the term 'Access, Equity and Inclusion' nor mention RRI/RI. But AEI has much relevance for STI policies and can be used by policy makers in addressing specific issues (Srinivas 2020) (Table 3.1).

The AEI framework must be developed further to contextualize RRI in India and elsewhere. Tools to measure Access, Equity and Inclusion are needed. The theoretical framework also must be made robust. While RRI is focused on formal innovations or innovations in the organized sector, new models of innovations like frugal innovation, inclusive innovation and grassroots innovation have taken shape, particularly in India. In the global South these are important forms of innovation that are not well understood or explained in terms of typical approaches to innovation. In both theory and practice India has contributed significantly on these. They do not challenge the idea of RRI but rather show that innovation can arise in different contexts and for different needs. There are significant lessons for RRI discourse and practice

Table 3.1 AEI in relation to RRI Keys, STIP 2020 (DRAFT) and RRI

Key	Overview	STIP 2020 DRAFT	Notes	RRI policy and discourse
Access (*Corresponding RRI Key: Open Access/Open Science, Governance*)	Access broadly defined covers access to basic needs including education. In RRI Open Access and Governance are relevant for access	Thrust on Open Science, Sharing of facilities in S&T institutions, National Research Foundation, Plan for access to journal articles	Access to innovations is an issue not limited to India. Access can be legitimized from the Right to Enjoy Benefits of Science	Open Science has been endorsed by European Commission. Many projects in RRI have focused on Open Science/Open Access and have come up with policy recommendations
Equity (*Corresponding RRI Key: Gender and Open Science and Governance*)	Equity covers equitable access, equity in distribution of benefits from innovation. Equity is not the same as equality	The focus in STIP is more on equity from a gender perspective than from integrating equity with STI. This evident in Chap. 7 which proposes many new approaches besides referring to Athena SWAN). But STIP limits equity mostly to gender and there too scope is limited as it does not discuss inclusive innovations for women nor approaches equity in STI as a major issue to be addressed	Equity in STI has been discussed in the context of technologies as well as a general principle (Srinivas 2020)	Gender in STI has been supported through projects on this, emphasis on Open Science and in public engagement in science which as an equity aspect. Governance in RRI is broad and offers scope for bringing an equity perspective to STI

(continued)

from these, but these will not be elaborated here for reasons of space. As pointed out earlier, although these may pose challenges to a narrow conception of RRI that excludes such innovations and prioritizes only innovation that arises from R&D in organized/formal sectors, this can be addressed by contextualizing RRI and by enriching RRI in theory and practice. In this, India can play an important role.

Table 3.1 (continued)

Key	Overview	STIP 2020 DRAFT	Notes	RRI policy and discourse
Inclusion (*Corresponding RRI Keys: Public Engagement, Open Science and Ethics*)	Inclusion implies inclusion of different stakeholders as beneficiaries and participants. An ethical framework that includes the concerns of different stakeholders is an inclusive framework	Inclusion is addressed by programs that provide specific quotas and preferences in education, jobs and access to services. STIP's chapter on Equity & Inclusion covers inclusion but it is a limited one. STIP touches upon Public Engagement, gives importance to Open Science and pays little attention to ethics. So, its approach towards inclusion is partial and problematic	Inclusion enhances the legitimacy of STI and enriches STI in theory and practice. Ethics provides the moral compass and ensures that in the name of STI socially acceptable boundaries are not crossed	RRI promotes public engagement, citizen science and other means to bring science and society closer and promotes greater stakeholder engagement. In that sense inclusion lies at the core of RRI

Vasen (2017) has identified five issues that have to be considered for making the RRI framework more relevant in developing countries, particularly in Latin America. In my view, a similar analysis for making RRI more relevant for India can be undertaken. Bigger developing countries like China, India, and Brazil are also major innovators and hence making RRI relevant in them is a challenge as well as an opportunity for making RRI more meaningful and useful. According to Yangdong et al. (2018),RRI has an affinity with the five development concepts in China, i.e., innovation, coordination, green development, opening up, and sharing. They point that RRI has been written into the 13th Five Year Plan for Science Technology and Innovation and that cultural tradition, development stage, and social structure should be considered when implementing RRI in China. In the case of India this exercise can benefit from studies done in India on RRI and RI (e.g., Chaturvedi et al. 2016, Mishra and Singh 2018). The Indian versions of RRI and RI can emerge by contextualizing RRI and RI, taking into account a dialog with ideas like Scientific Temper, SSR, and the AEI framework, and case studies on grass roots innovations, inclusive innovations and frugal innovations. These versions can in fact draw upon the policy frameworks that have elements of RRI and RI.

Another stream that can contribute to this is research on RRI at a few institutions such as Research and Information System for Developing Countries and the Centre for Studies in Science Policy (CSSP) of Jawaharlal Nehru University. The former is a think tank actively working on RRI while the latter as an educational and research center is promoting RRI through research and education.

3.4 Conclusion

RRI as a concept and practice originated in Europe and with the active support of the EC it has gained much traction in the last decade and a half. It has not become a fad in innovation studies or STI policy, but has gained firm footing in policy and research although it is not yet mainstream. The heart of RRI lies in connecting science with society and developing a social contract for STI so that stakeholders participate and engage with STI as active citizens rather than as passive consumers or sceptical observers. For this, the six keys of RRI and AIRR principles provide the direction. The literature shows that despite criticisms and shortcomings in implementation the rationale and relevance of RRI is well accepted. Although it has been tested and implemented more in Europe than elsewhere, its relevance and scope for contextualization and adoption/adaptation elsewhere, particularly in the Global South has been raised in the literature. RRI has not been institutionalized in the Global South and is gaining traction.

This chapter has taken India as an example and I have argued that RRI can be contextualized and adapted in India. The STI policy under consideration, while not mentioning RRI/RI, gives importance to some of the RRI keys (Open Science, Gender and Science Education). At the same time concepts such as Access, Equity and Inclusion and Scientific Temper which are from India can enrich RRI theory and practice. Through mutual learning and dialogue, the scope for this can be explored further. As there is an increase in interest on RRI in/for Global South the time is ripe to engage in this.

3.5 Disclosures and Disclaimers

(1) I am with Research and Information System for Developing Countries (RIS), as a Senior Fellow & Consultant. RIS has been a partner in three RRI projects (ProGRESS, RRI Practice and NewHoRRIzon). I have benefitted much by participating in them. This chapter does not reflect the views of these projects or RIS. It is written in my personal capacity, and it is not an output or part of any deliverable from any of those projects. I have cited and referred to literature from the two projects (i.e. RRI Practice and NewHoRRIzon).

(2) I have done a peer review of a version of STIP for DST and otherwise I have nothing to do with STIP or the process that resulted in the version of STIP I

reviewed. In other words, I have not been associated with the preparation of the STIP version (Department of Science and Technology DST 2020) reviewed by me or with the STIP process in any capacity or in any manner. At the time of writing (July 2022) STIP has not been officially announced. Nor there is an official announcement that it will be adopted and implemented with effect from a specific date. It is presumed that there will be a STI Policy as an outcome of the STIP process and this chapter is written with that presumption.

References

Abraham, Itty. 2021a. The two faces of India's new science and tech policy. https://science.thewire.in/the-sciences/india-national-research-foundation-draft-stip-2020-science-and-technology-policy-review/. Accessed 17 May 2021a.

Abraham, Itty. 2021b. Why 2003 was an important year for India's S&T policy resolutions. https://science.thewire.in/the-sciences/why-2003-was-an-important-year-for-indias-st-policy-resolutions/. Accessed 18 May 2021b.

Asveld, Lotte, and Rietje van Dam-Mieras. 2018. Introduction: Responsible research and innovation for sustainability. In *Responsible Innovation 3: A European Agenda*, ed. Lotte Asveld and Rietje van Dam-Mieras, 1–8. Heidelberg: Springer.

Beumer, Koen. 2019. Nation-building and the governance of emerging technologies: the case of nanotechnology in India. *NanoEthics* 13: 5–19. https://doi.org/10.1007/s11569-018-0327-8.

Bhaduri, Saradindu, and Nazia Talat. 2020. RRI beyond its comfort zone: initiating a dialogue with frugal innovation by 'the vulnerable.' *Science, Technology & Society* 25: 273–290. https://doi.org/10.1177/0971721820902967.

Braun Robert, Robert Gianni and Krishna Ravi Srinivas. 2020. *Policy Transfer and Shared Knowledge Base Learning from Policy Implementation Responsible Research and Innovation (RRI) in the European Union and Scientific Social Responsibility (SSR) in India.* NewHoRRIzon Project. https://newhorrizon.eu/wp-content/uploads/2020/04/NewHoRRIzon-Policy-Brief-3.pdf. Accessed 18 May 2021.

Chaturvedi, Sachin, and Krishna Ravi Srinivas. 2015. Science and technology for socio-economic development and quest for inclusive growth: emerging evidence from india. In *Science and technology governance and ethics a global perspective from europe, India and china*, ed. Miltos Ladikas, Sachin Chaturvedi, Yangdo Zhao, and Dirk Stemerding, 83–98. Berlin: Springer.

Chaturvedi, Sachin, Krishna Ravi Srinivas, and Amit Kumar. 2016. Agricultural technology choices and the RRI framework: emerging experiences from China and India. *Asian Biotechnology and Development Review* 18 (1): 93–111.

Christensen, Malene Vinther, Mika Nieminen, Marlene Altenhofer, Elise Tancoigne, Niels Mejlgaard, Erich Griessler, and Adolf Filacek. 2020. What's in a name? Perceptions and promotion of responsible research and innovation practices across Europe. *Science and Public Policy* 47 (3): 360–370. https://doi.org/10.1093/scipol/scaa018.

Coenen, Christopher. 2016. Broadening discourse on responsible research and innovation (RRI). *NanoEthics* 10: 1–4.

Doezema, Tess, David Ludwig, Phil Macnaghten, Clare Shelley-Egan, and Ellen-Marie Forsberg. 2019. Translation, transduction, and transformation: expanding practices of responsibility across borders. *Journal of Responsible Innovation* 6 (3): 323–331.

Department of Science and Technology DST. 1983. *Technology Policy Statement*. New Delhi: DST. http://www.nstmis-dst.org/TPStatement.aspx. Accessed 10 July 2021.

Department of Science and Technology DST. 2003. *Science and Technology Policy*. New Delhi: DST. https://indiabioscience.org/media/articles/STP-2003.pdf. Accessed 10 July 2021.

Department of Science and Technology DST. 2013. *Science, Technology and Innovation Policy*. New Delhi: DST. http://dst.gov.in/sites/default/files/STI%20Policy%202013-English.pdf. Accessed 10 July 2021.

Department of Science and Technology DST. 2020. *Science, Technology and Innovation Policy (Draft)*. New Delhi: DST. https://dst.gov.in/sites/default/files/STIP_Doc_1.4_Dec2020.pdf. Accessed 10 July 2021.

Department of Science and Technology DST. 2022. *Scientific Social Responsibility (SSR) Guidelines*. New Delhi: DST. https://dst.gov.in/sites/default/files/SSR%20Guidelines%202022%20Book_0.pdf. Accessed 10 July 2021.

European Commission. 2004. *Responsible research and innovation: Europe's ability to respond to societal challenges*. Brussels: European Commission.

European Commission. 2020a. *Institutional changes towards responsible research and innovation–achievements in horizon 2020 and recommendations on the way forward*. Brussels: European Commission Directorate-General for Research and Innovation.

Department of Science and Technology. 2020. Scientific Social Responsibility (SSR). (Draft) New Delhi: Department of Science and Technology.

European Commission. 2020b. *Responsible Research and Innovation*. Brussels: European Commission https://ec.europa.eu/programmes/horizon2020b/en/h2020-section/responsible-research-innovation. Accessed 18 May 2021.

Fisher, Erik. 2020. Reinventing responsible innovation. *Journal of Responsible Innovation* 7 (1): 1–5. https://doi.org/10.1080/23299460.2020.1712537.

Gao, Lu., Miao Liao, and Yandong Zhao. 2019. Exploring complexity, variety and the necessity of RRI in a developing country: the case of China. *Journal of Responsible Innovation* 6 (3): 368–374. https://doi.org/10.1080/23299460.2019.1603572.

Geoghegan-Quinn, Máire. 2012. *Commissioner Geoghegan-Quinn keynote speech at the 'Science in Dialogue' Conference Odense*, 23–25 April 2012. http://ec.europa.eu/archives/commission-2010-2014/geoghegan-quinn/headlines/speeches/2012/documents/20120423-dialogue-conference-speech_en.pdf. Accessed 18 May 2021.

Government of India. 1958. *Scientific policy resolution*. New Delhi: Government of India. https://indiabioscience.org/media/articles/SPR-1958.pdf. Accessed 10 July 2021.

Hartley, Sarah, Carmen McLeod, Mike Clifford, Sarah Jewitt, and Charlotte Ray. 2019. A retrospective analysis of responsible innovation for low-technology innovation in the Global South. *Journal of Responsible Innovation* 6 (2): 143–162.

Indian Council of Medical Research (ICMR). 2017. *National Ethical Guidelines for Biomedical and Health Research Involving Human Participants*. New Delhi: ICMR.

Jakobsen, Stig-Erik., Arnt Fløysand, and John Overton. 2019. Expanding the field of responsible research and innovation (RRI)—from responsible research to responsible innovation. *European Planning Studies* 27 (12): 2329–2343.

Krishna, Veni Venkata. 2013. Science, technology and innovation policy 2013: high on goals, low on commitment. *Economic and Political Weekly* 48 (16): 15–19.

Mahanti, Subodh. 2013. A perspective on scientific temper in india. *Journal of Scientific Temper* 1 (1&2): 46–62.

Mei, Liang, Hannot Rodríguez, and Jin Chen. 2020. Responsible innovation in the contexts of the European union and china: differences, challenges and opportunities. *Global Transitions* 2: 1–3.

Mishra, Shilpa, and Rajbeer Singh. 2018. Responsible innovation: a new approach to address the theoretical gaps for innovating in emerging E-mobility sector. In *Governance and Sustainability of Responsible Research and Innovation Processes,* eds. Fernando Ferri, Ned Dwyer, Saša Raicevich, Patrizia Grifoni, Husne Altiok, Hans Thor Andersen, Yiannis Laouris, and Cecilia Silvestri, 93–99. Amsterdam: Springer.

Ministry of Finance 2017. Economic survey: 2017–18. Department of economic affairs. Ministry of Finance, Government of India.

Jawahar Lal Nehru. 1946 Reprinted (1981). The Discovery of India. New Delhi: Jawaharlal Nehru Memorial Fund & Oxford University Press.

NITI Aayog. 2017. *S&T Vision 2032*. New Delhi: NITI Aayog.

Novitzky, Peter, Michael J. Bernstein, Vincent Blok, Robert Braun, Tung Chan, Wout Lamers, Anne Loeber, Ingeborg Meijer, Ralf Lindner, and Erich Griessler. 2020. Improve alignment of research policy and societal values. *Science* 369 (6499): 39–41. https://doi.org/10.1126/science.abb3415.

Nucleus Project. 2017. *RRI in China and South Africa: cultural adaptation report*. Deliverable 3.3. https://research.utwente.nl/en/publications/rri-in-china-and-south-africa-cultural-adaptation-report-delivera. Accessed 18 May 2021.

ORBIT. No date. *The keys of responsible research and innovation*. https://www.orbit-rri.org/resources/keys-of-rri/. Accessed 18 May 2021.

Ortt, Roland, I.R. van de Poel, D.C. van Putten, and L.M. Kamp. 2020. Introduction: exploring responsible innovation of large technological systems in society. In *Responsible innovation in large technological systems*, eds. J. Roland Ortt, David van Putten, Linda M. Kamp, and Ibo van de Poel, 1–17. New York: Routledge.

Owen, Richard, Ellen-Mary Forsberg, and Clare Shelley-Egan. 2019. *RRI-practice policy recommendations and roadmaps*, RRI-practice project report. Deliverable 16.2. www.rri-practice.eu/wp-content/uploads/2019/06/RRI-Practice_Policy_recommendations.pdf. Accessed 18 May 2021.

Owen, Richard, René von Schomberg, and Phil Macnaghten. 2021. An unfinished journey? Reflections on a decade of responsible research and innovation. *Journal of Responsible Innovation* 8 (2): 217–233. https://doi.org/10.1080/23299460.2021.1948789.

Pingali, Prabhu. 2012. Green revolution: toward 2.0. In *Proceedings of the National Academy of Sciences* 109(31):12302–12308. doi: https://doi.org/10.1073/pnas.0912953109.

Scholten, Bruce A. 2010. *India's white revolution: operation flood, food aid and development*. London: Bloomsbury.

Setiawan, Andri Dwi. 2018. *Responsible innovation: from concept to application: cases of energy technology adoption in Indonesia*. Eindhoven: Technische Universiteit Eindhoven. https://research.tue.nl/en/publications/responsible-innovation-from-concept-to-application-cases-of-energ. Accessed 18 May 2021.

Smith, Robert, Deborah Scott, Thoko Kamwendo, and Jane Calvert. 2019. *An Agenda for Responsible Research and Innovation in ERA* CoBioTech. Swindon, UK: Biotechnology and Biological Sciences Research Council and ERA CoFund on Biotechnology.

Srinivas, Krishna Ravi, Amit Kumar, and Nimita Pandey. 2018. *Report from National Case study: India*. Deliverable 11.1. https://www.rri-practice.eu/wp-content/uploads/2018/09/RRI-Practice_National_Case_Study_Report_INDIA.pdf. Accessed 18 May 2021.

Srinivas, Krishna Ravi. 2020. RIS Policy Brief 94 Access, equity and inclusion and science, technology and innovation policy New Delhi: RIS https://www.ris.org.in/sites/default/files/Publication/Policy%20brief-94%20Dr%20Ravi%20K%20Srinivas.pdf

Srinivas, Krishna Ravi, and Poonam Pandey. 2019. Indian perspectives on responsible innovation. In *Handbook on responsible innovation*, ed. Rene von Schomberg and Jonathan Hankins, 455–473. Cheltenham: Edward Elgar Publishing.

Stilgoe, Jack, Richard Owen, and Phil Macnaghten. 2013. Developing a framework for responsible innovation. *Research Policy* 42 (9): 1568–1580.

Valkenburg, Govert, Annapurna Mamidipudi, Poonam Pandey, and Wiebe E. Bijker. 2020. Responsible innovation as empowering ways of knowing. *Journal of Responsible Innovation* 7 (1): 6–25.

Van den Hoven, Jeroen. 2017. *Responsible innovation in brief*. https://d2k0ddhflgrk1i.cloudfront.net/TBM/Over%20faculteit/Afdelingen/Values%2C%20Technology%20and%20Innovation/People/Full%20Professors/Responsible_Innovation_in_brief.pdf. Accessed 18 May 2021.

Vasen, Federico. 2017. Responsible innovation in developing countries: an enlarged agenda. In *Responsible innovation 3, A European agenda*, ed. Lotte Asveld, Rietje van Dam-Mieras, Tsjalling Swierstra, Saskia Lavrijssen, Kees Linse, and Jeroen van den Hoven, 93–109. Heidelberg: Springer.

Von Schomberg, Rene. 2011. *Towards responsible research and innovation in the information and communication technologies and security technologies fields*. Luxembourg: Publications Office of the European Union. https://data.europa.eu/doi/10.2777/58723. Accessed 18 May 2021.

Wakunuma, Kutoma, Fabio de Castro, Tilimbe Jiya, Edurne A. Inigo, Vincent Blok, and Vincent Bryce. 2021. Reconceptualising responsible research and innovation from a Global South perspective. *Journal of Responsible Innovation* 8 (2): 267–291. https://doi.org/10.1080/23299460.2021.1944736.

Yan, Ping, and Wim Ravesteijn. 2019. Chinese road to responsible innovation: constructing a green port in Dalian. *WIT Transactions on The Built Environment* 187:109–119. https://www.witpress.com/elibrary/wit-transactions-on-the-built-environment/187/37367. Accessed 18 May 2021.

Yangdong, Zhao, Zhang Wenxia, Liao Miao, Huang Lei, Teng Fei, Song Runjie, Wu Yue, and Yao Yu. 2018. Report from National Case Study: China. RRI Practice Project. https://www.rri-practice.eu/wp-content/uploads/2018/09/RRI-Practice_National_Case_Study_Report_CHINA.pdf

Chapter 4
Formulating National Standards for Research Ethics Support and Review: The UKRIO/ARMA Case

John Oates

Abstract This chapter describes and analyses the background to and development of a national guidance framework for research ethics review that was commissioned by the United Kingdom Research Integrity Office and the Association of Research Managers and Administrators, and launched in 2020. Unlike the centrally-controlled UK Health Research Authority research ethics review system for health and social care research, ethics review of research outside these fields is not nationally controlled and is conducted within a wide variety of organisational structures. The development process had to adopt an approach that consulted widely and sought to ensure broad take-up of the guidance by offering a flexible approach to compliance with a set of superordinate principles, while meeting the expectations of the government funding body for the higher education sector as well as those of the UK research councils.

Keywords Research ethics review · Guidelines · Framework · Standards · UKRIO/ARMA

4.1 Introduction

Consistency, competence, and high standards are generally accepted as being the sine qua non for the review of research ethics protocols by research ethics committees (RECs). Until the early 2000s, the primary research ethics review activities in the United Kingdom (UK) were focused on a set of committees mostly concerned with medical research, under the auspices of the National Health Service (NHS), and a few newly formed within universities. But as such committees proliferated in the UK outside of the field of medical research, mainly in universities and in some charities and independent research organisations, there was little in the way of coordination and integration. Many different models of ethics review processes sprang up and concerns began to arise about the implications of such a totally decentralised and diverse system for the quality of reviews across the sector. The Association of

J. Oates (✉)
School of Education, Childhood and Youth Studies, The Open University, Milton Keynes, UK
e-mail: john.oates@open.ac.uk

© The Author(s) 2022
D. O'Mathúna and R. Iphofen (eds.), *Ethics, Integrity and Policymaking*, Research Ethics Forum 9, https://doi.org/10.1007/978-3-031-15746-2_4

49

Research Ethics Committees (AREC), initially established for chairs and secretaries of NHS RECs, welcomed members from these newly formed RECs and became a forum for exploring ways of building a set of common standards, paralleling the operating procedures already coordinating the NHS RECs. Work by a panel of AREC members, informed by discussions in a universities' forum also established by AREC, resulted in a guidance document launched in 2013 (Association of Research Ethics Committees (AREC) 2013). This document was well received by the sector. Increasing interest in being able to audit and document compliance with national expectations around research integrity led to the United Kingdom Research Integrity Office (UKRIO) and the Association of Research Administrators and Managers (ARMA) commissioning the development of national guidance based on the experience of institutions engaging with the AREC framework and the increasingly explicit expectations of research funding bodies for robust ethics review processes as part of a growing agenda around research integrity. The success of the AREC framework rested on its development in close liaison with the 'grassroots' of committee chairs, administrators and researchers as well as with the higher echelons of other stakeholders such as the major funding bodies. Led by a team including authors of the AREC document, the project to develop the UKRIO/ARMA guidance followed this approach to aim for the maximum buy-in by researchers and research institutions while also meeting the needs of funding and regulatory bodies in the UK.

4.2 Background

In 1991 the British Department of Health (DoH) formally established research ethics committees (RECs) in England to review proposed medical research projects, projects which were predominantly clinical trials of investigational medicinal products (CTIMPs) and trials of therapeutic approaches within the NHS. These committees were called Local Research Ethics Committees (LRECs). The establishment of LRECs in Wales and Scotland followed shortly afterwards.

With an increase in research involving more than one local area, multi-centre RECs (MRECs) were established in 1997 to review research proposals involving four or more local NHS areas. Responding to a need to continue to harmonise and standardise practice across all the RECs, the Central Office for Research Ethics Committees (COREC) was set up in 2000.

In consequence, there were many RECs across England, Scotland and Wales reviewing research proposals, with broadly similar structures and modes of operating. The Department of Health gave financial support to the independently formed AREC, which was incorporated as a limited company in 2002 initially as a forum primarily for chairs and secretaries of RECs to collaborate in considering issues in medical research ethics and the review practices of their committees. An important forum for developing this collaboration was established by the initiation of national conferences which tended on each occasion to focus on a specific research ethics topic, but also served as a valuable means for members of the Association to network and to build and maintain its 'community of practice'.

Outside of the medical and health research field, ethics review for other research with humans was not widely available around this time. By far the greater part of such research was carried out by researchers in universities. While some universities had well-founded RECs that had been operating successfully for some time, others had only embryonic systems or none at all. The lack of a coordinated national approach was highlighted in a King's College London survey carried out in 2003–4 (Tinker and Coomber 2004). This found that of the 87 universities that responded (out of 115 contacted) only two in five had any form of ethics review that had been in place for more than four years, and one in five had no processes for ethics scrutiny at all. While this survey documented a rapidly increasing awareness in universities of the need for universal scrutiny of research with humans, it also showed great variation in practice, with some universities having opted for a centralised model yet with others having devolved responsibility for ethics review to departmental levels.

The National Research Ethics Service (NRES) was founded by the DoH in 2007, bringing together COREC, MRECs and LRECs under a common umbrella body, with the aim of further standardising review practices under a common governance framework.

As the membership of AREC grew, by 2007 the Association had developed working collaborations both within and beyond the UK. In the UK, productive links were established with Universities UK, the United Kingdom Research Integrity Office (UKRIO) and with NRES, and links were strengthened with the DoH, inputting into new developments in ethics review including the Integrated Research Application System. Beyond the UK, connections were made with EUREC, the European network of RECs, and the European Forum of Good Clinical Practice. Drawing on the 'grass-roots' experience of reviewing a wide range of research proposals across nations, AREC was able to influence the development of policies and practices from a sound evidence base, as well as working within the Association to iron out differences between RECs in the interest of fostering common best practice standards.

The King's College survey of research ethics review of human research projects outside of the medical and health field highlighted a stark contrast between the two sectors and AREC welcomed a large influx of members from the university sector as awareness grew of the increasing concern with research ethics by funders and other stakeholders (Tinker and Coomber 2004). Work began towards the encouragement and development of high-quality REC practice in this sector. An important development at this time was the setting-up by AREC members of a Universities Ethics Forum, an informal space where people involved with university RECs could share experiences much as the prior membership of AREC had been encouraging. Views expressed in this forum, and discussions at an AREC conference, led to a working group of AREC members coming together to draw on universities' practices to develop an initial guidance document to set some common standards and principles, and to contribute further towards building better coherence and uniformity of research ethics review in the UK higher education sector. The working group brought together a wide range of experience in different universities and in different roles within governance and ethics review structures.

4.3   The Case Study

4.3.1   First Steps: The AREC Framework

The challenge faced in this project was presented by the great diversity of approach and practice in the sector at the time. In part, this diversity had arisen because the development of REC systems had been taken forward at the level of individual institutions which differed greatly in the volume and types of research with humans carried out within them, and the location of the research within their structures. As well as this diversity, governance structures varied and the governance locations and management lines within which RECs could sit also affected how reviewing was carried out and overseen. For example, a university with a very active research area in psychology was likely to have a departmental level committee dealing with both staff and students' research, while a university with less human-based research spread across several faculties was more likely to have a higher-level REC handling applications for review. Some universities had a high-level ethics committee that rarely reviewed applications but rather set policy and oversaw the reviewing of several departmental level RECs, while others had a single REC handling all reviewing. It was clear to the working group that a 'one-size-fits-all', such as was largely the case with NHS RECs, was not going to be feasible or practical in meeting the varied needs of this range of institutional structures and disciplinary specialisms.

The solution adopted by the working group was to concentrate on developing a framework that had sufficient flexibility to be able to accommodate this range of variation within universities but at the same time to provide common standards and an audit tool to allow for evidencing compliance with these common standards (Association of Research Ethics Committees (AREC) 2013). At an early stage, a set of four guiding principles was proposed and elaborated, a novel development given that there had been no such explicit principles for ethics review in existence previously, even though principles for ethical research conduct have a clear and very long history.

The first principle, *independence*, was established as a basic requirement for a REC to be able to deliberate in its evaluations of research ethics protocols without conflicts of interest. This stresses the need for reviewers to have sufficient distance from the researchers applying for review to enable them to undertake a balanced, objective analysis of the risks and potential harms in a research proposal and the adequacy of the researchers' plans to eliminate or at least minimise and mitigate the risks. Clearly, ethics review by academic members of a department where the same members are also colleagues of researchers applying for review would not meet this criterion, yet at the time of elaborating this principle there were indeed ethics reviews being conducted with just this flaw.

But independence alone does not guarantee a good, thorough, and well-informed ethics review. It needs to be complemented by the application of the second principle, *competence*. As well as ensuring that those reviewing cases have adequate experience and knowledge, a well-founded REC needs clear operating procedures and terms of reference, for which the working group developed a set of recommendations, based on what consultations with REC chairs and administrators identified as best practice at that time.

The working group also intended the review principles to help RECs overcome and indeed change what was a dominant view, that ethics review was a hurdle to be overcome and then put behind as the research progressed. Instead, the group wished to promote *facilitation* as the third core principle; that seeking an ethics review should come to be seen by researchers as a positive component of their research process, one that could enhance the quality of their work rather than merely 'police' it and avoid the common charge of being 'obstructive'.

Finally, to counter another common view, that the workings of RECs were obscure and hidden, with the reasons for decisions not being clear, the fourth principle, *openness*, was intended to promote practices of transparency, such as keeping clear records of decision-making and making explicit the reasons for decisions when these are communicated to applicants.

Following discussion of these principles in a workshop associated with the 2009 AREC national conference, the group then engaged in a period of consultations with a range of stakeholders, with funding bodies such as the Economic and Social Research Council (ESRC), with the Health Research Authority (the body responsible for the ethics review of medical research), with Universities UK and through a number of joint actions with learned societies in the social sciences through the Academy of Social Sciences.

To help to ensure alignment across the social sciences, members of the working group engaged with parallel developments in guidance, codes and practices for ethical research conduct underway in bodies including the ESRC, the British Psychological Society and the Social Research Association. The AREC universities research ethics forum proved to be a further crucial consultation mechanism, especially in relation to the feasibility of the structural and process guidance being developed. A Universities Development Group, which emerged naturally as the AREC forum became a source for sharing ideas for best practice, played an additional collaborative role in ensuring alignment with governance developments in universities.

A further parallel development, by Universities UK (UUK), was the consultation on the first Concordat on Research Integrity, which had similar high-level aims to the AREC project in seeking to support common standards of best practice in research integrity. Integrity and ethics share common ground, and the Concordat recognised the role of the university sector's REC review processes as an element of research integrity. Members of the AREC group contributed to the consultation on the Concordat, which was published in 2012 (UUK 2012). The self-assessment tool, an audit framework, which the AREC group had developed, nicely helped to serve the new reporting requirements of the Concordat.

The extensive co-production process finally led to the publication in 2013 of the AREC Framework of Policies and Procedures for University Research Ethics Committees (Association of Research Ethics Committees (AREC) 2013), promoted by AREC as a set of guidelines to help higher education institutions develop their research ethics review policies, structures, and procedures.

4.3.2 Second Steps: UKRIO/ARMA Guidance

Recognising the increased interest that the university sector was showing in seeking guidance on research ethics, senior officers in UKRIO and ARMA decided that a further useful step would be to build on the experience of the AREC framework, taking account of developments in the field, to produce an authoritative publication giving clear guidance on how best to manage research ethics review, not only for universities, but also for other research organisations. And, in addition, for this guidance to be aligned with the key principles of research integrity that were being promoted by the Concordat on Research Integrity, to support an open culture of auditing and reporting on institutional actions. A project team was formed, incorporating key members of the previous AREC working party as well as further representation across the research community. The team had useful links with other research ethics initiatives such as the revision of ethics codes of learned societies, ethics review within the Health Research Authority ambit, research councils' requirements for ethics review in the UK and ethics review practices in the European Research Council.

While the liaison and consultations that informed the AREC framework had been informal and largely opportunistic, the greater ambition for the UKRIO/ARMA guidance meant that formal processes of involvement with stakeholders were necessary not only for the adequate consideration of the relevant issues but also for the guidance to be perceived as being firmly grounded in the practicalities of research organisations' governance structures and processes, the criteria by which research integrity is scrutinised and the values and principles inherent in scientific research. To these ends, senior officials in UKRIO and ARMA established broad memberships of a steering and an advisory group, representing the necessary breadth of interests. Regular reporting and sharing of drafts with these two groups, and responding to their critical evaluations, while time-consuming, nevertheless led to a sense of shared ownership and hence willingness to adopt and endorse the final outputs.

Reflecting the greater engagement of universities with improving their processes around research ethics following the launch of the 2012 Concordat on Research Integrity, the UKRIO/ARMA project aimed to highlight the importance of building support for researchers throughout all stages of the research cycle. It sought to extend beyond the inevitably pre-emptive formal review carried out by RECs of protocols developed before the associated research data collection starts. With the proliferation of research methods in the social sciences, exploratory and co-produced research does not easily sit with reviews of ethics protocols before the ethics issues involved have been fully revealed, which is what a single engagement with a REC traditionally required. Nor does a lack of consultation with the expert knowledge held by REC members help with the preparatory phases of research when design and methods are being planned.

An early stage in the development of the new guidance was to validate the four basic principles for ethics review that had initially been proposed as the core of the AREC framework, by testing them with the advisory and steering groups, to see if they still held up in the new research environment. No challenges to them were expressed and it was recognised that working from such 'top-level' principles was an important feature, allowing them to be implemented flexibly across a range of different research organisations' structures.

Another key element, providing research organisations with a common, structured approach to auditing and reporting externally on ethics review, was the provision of a self-assessment tool. This had been a successful part of the AREC framework, and it was important to ensure that such a tool would be compliant with the expectations of the Concordat on Research Integrity for annual reporting to the Higher Education Funding Council for England. Again, input from the advisory and steering groups was vital here. The development of the second version of the Concordat went forward in parallel with the development of the new UKRIO/ARMA guidance and engaging with the professional network around this topic was instrumental in keeping alignment.

The authoring team made a joint decision that it was important to draw out and make explicit the underlying rationale for the guidance to be offered. This resulted in a very extensive first full draft of 45 pages (more than 13,000 words). While this led to a rich dialogue as the consultation on this draft proceeded, comments were beginning to be made that it was looking like a somewhat 'unwieldy' document for its intended use. As well as comments from the steering and advisory groups, reactions were sought from a wide range of academics and administrators involved with research ethics. Members of the authoring team had been instrumental in taking forward the Academy of Social Sciences 'Generic Ethics Principles in Social Sciences' project (2013) which ran from 2010 to 2016. This project, while focused on principles for ethical research conduct, also included critical discussions of the processes of ethics review and evidenced acceptance of the four core principles for review first set out in the AREC framework. This project also generated a social network that proved to be of great value in garnering comment and support for the UKRIO/ARMA work.

On the completion of the second draft, building on comments from the initial consultations, its size had grown even more and discussions within the team could have easily become polarised due to conflicting comments coming through from the consultation; some praising the thoroughness of treatment and welcoming the full justification of the approach, while others were reacting in a totally opposite way, saying how a much briefer, concise document was needed, simply setting in clear terms 'how to do' ethics review. Some of the key stakeholders commented that this was a 'deal-breaker'. Quite negative comments were being made that the guidance would not be well received and would not be recommended across the sector unless there was a radical rethink of the length. Although the team was wedded to the fuller treatment, in part because of the work that had gone into it, it was also realised that some potential users, pressed for time as many are, would not be prepared to 'wade through' the full document to get to the prescriptions it offered. Achieving a consensus and thus facilitating take-up was a crucial aim, so the team managed to find an eclectic solution by drawing an analogy with the 'quick-start guide' often supplied alongside a full operating manual for equipment. As the third and final draft was being prepared, taking in further comments, a parallel, heavily edited version was created, omitting much of the rationale and background material in the full version, halving its size. With the agreement of the steering and advisory groups, the two versions then went into production for web delivery and were launched simultaneously by UKRIO and ARMA on April 8th, 2020 (UKRIO/ARMA 2020).

4.4 Analysis

Because the ethics review of UK research in health and social care is subject to 'top-down' governance by the NHS Health Research Authority, compliance with well-defined standard procedures for all reviews is controlled. With no such overarching control mechanism for ethics review in other fields, procedural standards have by necessity been 'home-grown' by the research organisations, primarily universities. While, as described above, several initiatives within the sector have sought to bring about a degree of consistency, the autonomy of governance by the research organisations is widely respected and indeed guarded, meaning that compliance with common standards can only be by voluntary rather than enforced adherence. As far as the actual procedures for ethics review are concerned, change is relatively easy even if it takes time to go through the institutional processes necessary to approve or amend standard operating procedures. Structural changes, for example in how a REC fits within a governance framework, are typically more resistant to change, and dependent on the review cycles and changes in top-level management. But there are external pressures for compliance, notably from national funding bodies such as the Higher Education Funding Council for England and the UK research councils, which have expectations that need to be met for the maintenance of research integrity. International funding bodies such as the European Research Council also set requirements for ethics review of projects and programmes that they fund. These external pressures mean that the availability of national guidance is attractive to research organisations but at the same time it needs to be flexible and practicable for the variety of structures and processes across the sector.

For these reasons, it was crucial in developing the UKRIO/ARMA (2020) guidance that it be seen to be wanting to support shared values and expectations, working democratically with key stakeholders and gatekeepers. This meant that it was necessary to recognize expertise and to identify where it was located, so establishing the memberships of the steering and advisory groups, and ensuring that communications were clear and timely, and that deadlines for comments allowed sufficient time. These were key to success.

It was also important to develop the guidance as driven by a set of clearly specified principles, rather than by rigid prescriptions of processes and structures, to allow for their implementation in a variety of ways, adapted to the local circumstances of research organisations.

4.5 Lessons Learned

A key lesson learned from the extended development period for the UKRIO/ARMA documents was that to produce guidance that will be accepted and acted on must indeed take a long time. This is because consultation, indeed very wide consultation, is crucial to success. And there needs to be consultation throughout, not at solely a single point in the process. Comments must be seen to be acted on, and involvement of stakeholders in at least two draft stages helps to ensure that this is achieved and helps to keep them on board to spend the time critically evaluating drafts, knowing that their comments will be taken seriously.

Involving a wide range of commentators, across the potential users of the guidance and including those influential persons who would facilitate or impede adoption, is crucial to success. A lot of time was spent during the development period of this guidance making personal contact with commentators and encouraging them to stay involved. This was particularly important where disagreements arose, for example over the length of the guidance, and sharing the solution personally with the people who felt most strongly about this was key to gaining their support.

Finding the eclectic solution, to produce the summary and full version, was, on reflection, a vitally important final step. If the team had tried to compromise by 'watering down' the full version, trying to reach a compromise position, it is likely that no-one would have been fully satisfied. So the lesson here is to keep an open, creative mind, even when a project is well under way.

4.6 Implications and Recommendations for Policymakers

For policies to be effectively implemented in 'tight' governance structures, those who are responsible for the implementation need to be convinced of the value of the policies in addition to being subject to contractual imperatives and sanctions for non-implementation. A key aspect of a policy's value lies in the extent to which it is based on trustworthy research-based evidence. Arguably the same top-level criteria apply to the assessment of the ethical soundness of research as to its scientific rigour, and these criteria map well onto three of the core principles of ethics review that frame the UKRIO/ARMA guidance: independence, competence and transparency.

Facilitation is not applicable in the same way. If it is accepted that the integrity value of scientific research includes ethics as well as soundness of method, interpretation and claims, then policymakers evaluating research should be looking for evidence that the conduct and ethics review of a research project comply with these principles.

Thus, where significant ethics issues are evident in a piece of research being scrutinised, evaluators should be looking at least for a clear statement that a 'favourable opinion' was given on the research by a named REC (or Institutional Review Board (IRB) in the case of research ethics influenced by US terminology). While IRBs and UK Health Research Authority RECs are governed by national standard operating procedures, this is not necessarily the case for institutional RECs outside of these. Due diligence in such cases could usefully include checks on the research ethics pages of the relevant institution's website, looking for evidence of compliance with an ethics framework such as that of UKRIO/ARMA. Further guidance and support on evaluating the 'ethicality' of research can be found in the PRO-RES (https://pro res-project.eu/) website assets.

References

Academy of Social Sciences. 2015. Generic Ethics Principles for Social Science Research. https://www.acss.org.uk/developing-generic-ethics-principles-social-science/academy-adopts-five-eth ical-principles-for-social-science-research/. Accessed 16 July 2021.

Association of Research Ethics Committees (AREC). 2013. A Framework of Policies and Procedures for University Research Ethics Committees. https://arma.ac.uk/wp-content/uploads/2017/08/Framework-of-policies-and-procedures.pdf. Accessed 01 Sept 2021.

Tinker, Anthea, and Vera Coomber. 2004. *University Research Ethics Committees: Their Role, Remit and Conduct*. King's College London/Nuffield Foundation.

UKRIO/ARMA. 2020. Research Ethics Support and Review (full and summary versions). https://ukrio.org/news/new-guidance-research-ethics-support-and-review-in-research-organisations/. Accessed 16 July 2021.

Universities UK. 2012. *The Concordat to Support Research Integrity*, Universities UK, London.

Chapter 5
Data Protection in Croatia: An Indicator of Ethics Processes in Research Institutions

Zvonimir Koporc

Abstract The implementation of the European Union's (EU) General Data Protection Regulation (GDPR) in the Republic of Croatia did not include derogations for scientific research purposes at the national level except for official statistical purposes. Research has shown that the Croatian Personal Data Protection Agency (AZOP) received very few inquiries related to personal data protection from academic and research institutions in Croatia, both before and after GDPR, but received many general inquiries and non-research-related reports. This chap uses Croatia as a case study to assess two explanations for this: that data protection is managed well in Croatian research, or that potential ethics issues in research data protection are not sufficiently recognized. This chap summarizes research findings exploring these issues, the inferences that can be drawn, and lessons learned that could contribute to research ethics processes in other European Member States.

Keywords Data protection · General Data Protection Regulation (GDPR) · Croatian Personal Data Protection Agency (AZOP) · Data Protection Officer (DPO) · Ethics assessment

5.1 Introduction

Replacing the EU's previous Data Protection Directive (Directive 95/46/EC), enacted in October 1995, the new General Data Protection Regulation (EU) 2016/679 (GDPR) enforced on May 25, 2018, primarily aimed to provide individuals control over their personal data and at the same time to unify the regulation within the EU (EU 2016). The GDPR introduced new obligations and more significant sanctions when compared to the previous directive (EU 1995). The GDPR offers possible derogations (e.g. for Article 9) and may impose additional requirements when appointing a Data Protection Officer (DPO) (Article 37) or when conducting Data Protection

Z. Koporc (✉)
School of Medicine, Catholic University of Croatia, Zagreb, Croatia
e-mail: zvonimir.koporc@unicath.hr

© The Author(s) 2022
D. O'Mathúna and R. Iphofen (eds.), *Ethics, Integrity and Policymaking*, Research Ethics Forum 9, https://doi.org/10.1007/978-3-031-15746-2_5

Impact Assessments (DPIA) as per Article 35. In Croatia, to ensure full implementation of the General Data Protection Regulation, the Act on the Implementation of the General Data Protection Regulation (Official Gazette, No. 44/2018) was enacted on May 25, 2018. Unfortunately, derogations for scientific research purposes were not implemented on the national level in the Republic of Croatia, except for official Croatian statistical purposes (Article 33) (Parliament 2018b; Puljak et al. 2020).

This made the use of personal data for scientific research in Croatia even more challenging compared to other EU countries that implemented proposed derogations for scientific purposes (such as in the Republic of Austria) (Parliament 2018a; DSB 2018). To explore the impact and implementation of GDPR on science and research in the Republic of Croatia, a study was prepared in cooperation with the Croatian Personal Data Protection Agency (known as AZOP based on its Croatian name, Agencija za zaštitu osobnih podataka), which is a member of the European Data Protection Board (EDPB). At first, we wanted to explore the possible level of issues related to personal data protection and associated with science and research in Croatia. We searched for all reported cases to AZOP coming from academic and research institutions across Croatia. Our findings showed that from January 2015 till the end 2019, AZOP received only 37 requests about personal data protection related to the use of data for research purposes (Puljak et al. 2020). Taking account of a large number of research institutions in Croatia, and the explored time-frame of five years which included the period before and after the implementation of GDPR, this number appears surprisingly low. However, the number of general requests and non-research-related data breach requests reported to AZOP were much higher when compared to those coming from academic and research institutions across the Republic of Croatia.

5.2 Implementation

The full implementation of GDPR pushed the numbers of citizens' complaints to a higher level, showing a positive impact of GDPR on citizens' personal data protection awareness. However, we also detected that in many cases, citizens misinterpreted their rights as AZOP did not find a valid ground to initiate official administrative procedures which would follow reported cases from the side of citizens.

Nevertheless, the focus of our interest remained with the implementation of GDPR in scientific and academic institutions across Croatia. The question that sparked our interest was why such a low number of requests for opinion were addressed to AZOP from academic and research institutions. Is the situation related to personal data protection in the academic and research environment so good that no complaints were coming from that area? Do research institutions in Croatia have some perfect system when dealing with protecting personal data so that there was no need for official intervention from the side of AZOP which would follow some of those rare, reported requests related to the use of personal data for research purposes? In an environment where derogations of GDPR for scientific purposes were not sufficiently implemented at the Croatian national level and knowing that complexity of research under the GDPR increased (Quinn 2021), that probability appeared less likely. That is why we assumed that the possible explanation for that effect might be the low awareness of GDPR implications for research work conducted in academic and research institutions in Croatia. To resolve that puzzle, our next step was to explore whether the responsibilities of DPOs (EC 2021) were appropriately recognized in their institutions, what kind of support they could count on and from who, what kinds of problems they face in their working positions and whether they have additional opportunities for professional advancement and continuous education in the field of data protection. Importantly, we also wanted to explore the relationship between DPOs and Research Ethics Committees in institutions where such committees had been established.

5.3 Background

Previous studies had emphasized the lack of formal training and the nature of the broad discussion on ethics that may occur in the work of Research Ethics Committees (Sperling 2021) and the appearance of inconsistencies between ethics committees' reviews (Trace and Kolstoe 2017). Furthermore, other studies showed that the heterogeneity of opinions between ethics board members, especially when the protection of the institution's interests are questioned, may lead to poor relations and mistrust between ethics committees and researchers (Guillemin et al. 2012).

However, Ethics Committees in academic institutions are seen as a crucial control mechanism for keeping the research ethical. Considering the fast and rapid development of new technologies, and the exponential growth of personal data used for research purposes, the role of Ethics Boards and Committees appears more important than ever. Questions related to the use of personal data in scientific research are increasing, especially in the EU after implementing the GDPR. Since not all EU countries implemented derogations of GDPR for scientific purposes, issues related to personal data protection are often exhausting the capacities of Ethics Boards and Committees. Personal data protection is one of the fields which may lead to "ethics overkill", the term which relates to demanding unnecessary ethical requirements, even where compliance is not possible (Nature 2014). In a large Horizon 2020 grant applications system (Kinderlerer 2016) involvement of a large number of new expert evaluators is crucial to keep the evaluation procedure fair. Unfortunately, that may potentially lead to the opposite situation—an unfair implementation of the system. Simply due to inexperience, new experts may simply "tick the box" in situations where they are uncertain or not sufficiently knowledgeable on some questions related to ethics. In our recent retrospective study performed on more than 79,000 MSCA H2020 applications, we found that one of the most commonly identified ethics categories, both by applicants in their "ethics self-assessment" form and during the ethics review procedures performed by ethics experts, was the "protection of personal data" (De Waele et al. 2021).

For all issues related to personal data protection, after introducing the GDPR, ethics review boards may also rely on a newly mandated Data Protection Officer (DPO) (EDPS no date). Assuming that DPOs might face difficulties with the implementation of GDPR in their institutions, we were very interested in investigating how DPOs function in their institutions, to possibly detect any hurdles or obstacles which may influence their work and to explore the previously mentioned relationship between Ethics Boards or Committees and DPOs.

Evidently DPOs should continuously develop their skills and broaden their knowledge in the field of personal data protection to be able to fulfill all tasks and duties described in Article 39 of the GDPR. Still, the GDPR did not set any legal obligations for that, nor were such duties introduced as mandatory at the national level. Furthermore, Article 37, recital 5 of the GDPR, states that "the data protection officer shall be designated on the basis of professional qualities and, in particular, expert knowledge of data protection law and practices" (EU 2016). When speaking about science and research in Croatia, we indicated two possible problems in the ethics review process associated with the use of personal data protection for research purposes. First, there is no specific legal obligation for institutional Ethics Committees to consult DPOs in the process of granting approvals in matters related to personal data protection, and second, above the recommendation that the DPOs should be knowledgeable in the field of data protection and should continuously develop their knowledge and skills in that area, there is no obligatory legal requirement to require DPOs to constantly develop their skills and knowledge in data protection. At the time point when we conducted our survey on DPOs across the Republic of Croatia, we did not come across any publication which explored the quality of DPOs' work output and their support to institutions where they are appointed.

5.4   DPOs and Ethical Research

To explore the relationship between DPOs and Ethics Boards and to explore the current position of DPOs in institutions across Croatia, together with AZOP we prepared a research study based on a cross-sectional online survey which was then completed by more than 700 DPOs across the Republic of Croatia (Mladinić et al. 2021).

As first, our study showed that institutions in the Republic of Croatia did not appropriately use the time between the adoption of GDPR in 2016 until the enforcement in the May of 2018. Namely, our findings showed that the median time period DPOs served at some institution was 18 months. Considering that this research was conducted between November 2020 and March 2021, our findings led us to a clear and disappointing conclusion that the majority of DPOs were appointed after the enforcement of GDPR only because of the formal legal obligation set by GDPR. An even more disappointing finding was that most surveyed DPOs claimed that they had no or minimal previous knowledge in personal data protection. An unclear explanation of the "expert knowledge" which the DPO is required to understand (Article 37 of the GDPR) did not set any specific requirement to demonstrate that candidates for the position of DPO would possess sufficient knowledge in the field of personal data protection which would enable them to fulfil all duties and tasks set for the DPO according to the GDPR. Obviously, institutions used that vague GDPR definition to appoint the DPO according to their institutional, organizational needs based on available staff and not based on the appropriate institutional data protection strategies. That vague and unclear description of the GDPR Article 37 without clearly defined rules or potential penalties for appointment of DPOs who do not possess appropriate background knowledge and skills, allowed institutions to appoint anyone to the position of DPO. Without clear appointment parameters, institutions were able to appoint anyone as DPO, just to fulfil a legal obligation. We found that the majority (92%) of surveyed DPOs in our study (Mladinić et al. 2021) were already employed by their institutions when they were appointed as a DPO. Indeed, such an appointment strategy was the easiest solution for institutions.

To test DPOs' basic knowledge regarding personal data protection we set two basic questions: one to describe the difference between anonymization and pseudonymization and the second to appropriately select privacy policy items. Unfortunately, on the first question, around forty percent partially correct or completely wrong answers were given, while only twenty percent of the tested DPOs correctly selected all ten privacy policy items. Our findings correlate with previously published claims that DPOs do not possess any in-depth knowledge of how to apply the GDPR (Sidlauskas 2019).

In our research (Mladinić et al. 2021), only a small number of DPOs indicated a research or an educational institution as their employer. Even in that small sample, it was clear that they received just a few research-related questions which were in line with previously published data (Puljak et al. 2020; Dinu 2018). Surprisingly, most DPOs (59% of surveyed DPOs) did not receive any single request for an opinion or a single complaint regarding personal data processing from the side of citizens/responders. That was in contradiction with results from this same study showing a DPO's strong perception of a workload increase associated with the introduction of GDPR. Namely, even though only 36% of the surveyed DPOs responded to questions related to the changes induced by the GDPR, the most common answers were related to the increase in the workload, tasks and administration. Our research did not explore the specifics of the stated increase in workload, but their feeling of such additional workload may be associated with the fact that the majority of tested DPOs in our survey did not show basic knowledge about personal data protection, nor did they conduct basic processes related to personal data protection for which they were supposed to. We also found that most of the DPOs did not analyze personal data processing activities in their organization, and also, they did not conduct or participated in a data protection impact assessment.

Considering that most DPOs indicated that they could perform their work independently, it seems that most DPOs were not fully aware of their duties and responsibilities while serving as DPOs in their institutions.

5.5 DPOs and Ethics Committees

Furthermore, our study (Mladinić et al. 2021) showed that only around thirty percent of DPOs claimed to have an ethics committee in their institution where they worked. From those which indicated having an ethics committee in their institution, only a few DPOs received some official request or were contacted by their institutional ethics committee and the majority was not involved in that committee's work in any way. These results may indicate that from the one side, researchers rarely contact DPOs or Ethics Committees regarding questions related to data protection as they do not sufficiently recognize the ethical issues which may arise from the inappropriate implementation of the personal data protection. Furthermore, only a few DPOs were involved in institutional ethics committees, mainly as administrative support and only a few were involved as a committee member. One of the most worrying findings from our survey was that most of those DPOs did not know whether they were sufficiently competent to answer the potential questions of an ethics committee. Even though only 11% of those DPOs replied on our question about what might help them, their institutions or their Ethics Committees to increase their effectiveness and productivity in tasks related to personal data protection, their answers clearly pointed to the DPOs needing additional education.

5.6 Summary Conclusion

Our results point to the need for continuous education or continuous professional development (CPD) of DPOs and a better definition of "expert knowledge" needed for a DPO appointment. Furthermore, our study indicates the pressing need for CPD of DPOs in personal data protection and possibly some standardization in DPO education even though the GDPR does not prescribe the certification of the DPOs.

Such standardized DPO education might be based on a voluntary certification procedure that will include standardized and professional education conducted from the side of national data protection agencies. However, such voluntary certification would not mean that certification would be considered as an end-stage in the DPOs' education process; on the contrary, a DPO must continue in education since the personal data protection issues keep evolving with the development and introduction of new and previously unknown technologies (Hirsch et al. 2019).

Even though we consider that we solved one part of the puzzle in the relationship between the DPO and Ethics Committees, the second part of that riddle, with the emphasis on Ethics Committees' perceptions and potential problems which they face in the area of personal data protection in their ethics assessment procedures, especially after the introduction of GDPR, still remains to be answered in future research.

Finally, questions on how to reconcile the needs of usage of personal data for scientific research purposes together with the individuals' rights to preserve their rights related to personal data are coming to a critical time point. Clear guidance from the side of EC structures dealing with personal data protection or national governmental structures in this area is more than needed. Recognizing the need to help relevant stakeholders and to further clarify the application of the GDPR to the processing of personal data for scientific research purposes, on April 30, 2021, the EDPB organized a special remote stakeholder event (EDPB 2021). All this points to the need for further improvement and updating of the current GDPR version, especially in relation to the use of personal data in scientific purposes. Our work showed the need for further improvement of GDPR especially in relation to article 37 (*Designation of the data protection officer*) and article 89. Moreover, it seems that paragraph 2 of article 89 (*Safeguards and derogations relating to processing for archiving purposes in the public interest, scientific or historical research purposes or statistical purposes*) mentioning potential use of derogations which is given to the Member State law must be additionally encouraged and it might require further clarifications.

References

De Waele, I., D. Wizel, L. Puljak, and Z. Koporc. 2021. Ethics appraisal procedure in 79,670 marie skłodowska-curie proposals from the entire European HORIZON 2020 research and innovation program (2014–2020): A retrospective analysis. *PLoS ONE* 16 (11): e0259582. https://doi.org/10.1371/journal.pone.0259582.

Dinu, M.S. 2018. New data protection regulations and their impact on universities. In *Elearning Challenges and New Horizons,* Vol 4, eds. I. Roceanu, S. Topor, C. Holotescu, C. Radu, F. Nitu, G. Grosseck, and M. Radoi, 26–33. Bucharest: 'Carol I' National Defence University Publishing House.

DSB, Austrian Data Protection Authority. 2018. https://www.data-protection-authority.gv.at/data-protection-laws/relevant-data-protection-laws.html. Accessed 31 Dec 2021.

EC, European Commission. 2021. What are the responsibilities of a Data Protection Officer (DPO)? https://ec.europa.eu/info/law/law-topic/data-protection/reform/rules-business-and-org anisations/obligations/data-protection-officers/what-are-responsibilities-data-protection-off icer-dpo_en. Accessed 31 Dec 2021.

EDPB, European Data Protection Board. 2021. EDPB Stakeholder Event on processing of personal data for scientific research purposes. European Data Protection Board. https://edpb.europa.eu/news/news/2021/edpb-stakeholder-event-processing-personal-data-scientific-research-purpos es_en. Accessed 31 December 2021.

EDPS, European Data Protection Supervisor. No date. Data Protection Officer (DPO). https://edps.europa.eu/data-protection/data-protection/reference-library/data-protection-officer-dpo_en. Accessed 31 Dec 2021.

EU, The European Parliament and the Council. 1995. Directive 95/46/EC of the European Parliament and of the Council of 24 October 1995 on the protection of individuals with regard to the processing of personal data and on the free movement of such data. In *OJ L 281*: Official Journal of the European Union.

EU, The European Parliament and the Council. 2016. Regulation (EU) 2016/679 of the European parliament and of the Council of 27 April 2016 on the protection of natural persons with regard to the processing of personal data and on the free movement of such data, and repealing Directive 95/46/EC (General Data Protection Regulation). In *L 119/1*: Official Journal of the European Union.

Guillemin, M., L. Gillam, D. Rosenthal, and A. Bolitho. 2012. Human research ethics committees: examining their roles and practices. *Journal of Empirical Research on Human Research Ethics* 7 (3): 38–49. https://doi.org/10.1525/jer.2012.7.3.38.

Hirsch, Francois, Ron Iphofen, and Zvonimir Koporc. 2019. Ethics assessment in research proposals adopting CRISPR technology. *Biochemia Medica (zagreb)* 29 (2): 020202. https://doi.org/10.11613/bm.2019.020202.

Kinderlerer, J., and D. Schroeder. 2016. Assessment of the Ethics Appraisal Process of Horizon 2020. Director General DG-RTD, European Commission.

Mladinić, A., L. Puljak, and Z. Koporc. 2021. Post-GDPR survey of data protection officers in research and non-research institutions in Croatia: a cross-sectional study. *Biochemia Medica (zagreb)* 31 (3): 030703. https://doi.org/10.11613/bm.2021.030703.

Nature, Editorial. 2014. Ethical overkill. *Nature* 516 (7530): 143–144. https://doi.org/10.1038/516143b.

Parliament, Republic of Austria. 2018a. Federal Act concerning the Protection of Personal Data (DSG).

Parliament, Republic of Croatia. 2018b. Implementation of the general data protection regulation. *Official Gazette* 44/2018.

Puljak, Livia, Anamarija Mladinic, Ron Iphofen, and Zvonimir Koporc. 2020. Before and after enforcement of GDPR: Personal data protection requests received by Croatian Personal Data Protection Agency from Academic and Research Institutions. *Biochemia Medica (Zagreb)* 30(3). doi: https://doi.org/10.11613/bm.2020.030201.

Quinn, Paul. 2021. Research under the GDPR – a level playing field for public and private sector research? *Life Sciences, Society and Policy* 17 (1): 4. https://doi.org/10.1186/s40504-021-00111-z.

Sidlauskas, A. 2019. Opportunities for DPO (Data Protection Officer) occupational training and improvement. In *13th International Technology, Education and Development Conference*, ed. Chova, L.G., Martinez, A.L., and Torres, I.C. 808–814. Valenica: International Academy of Technology, Education and Development.

Sperling, D. 2021. "Like a sheriff in a small town": status, roles, and challenges of ethics committees in academic colleges of education. *Journal of Empirical Research on Human Research Ethics* 16: 290–303. https://doi.org/10.1177/15562646211005253.

Trace, S., and S.E. Kolstoe. 2017. Measuring inconsistency in research ethics committee review. *BMC MedIcal Ethics* 18 (1): 65. https://doi.org/10.1186/s12910-017-0224-7.

Chapter 6
Science Advisors and "Good Evidence": A Case Study

Gabi Lombardo

Abstract This chapter addresses the place of research ethics in evidence-informed policy and the role of those who are elevated to special roles to advise governments. Science advisors are one type of institutional link between scientific research and policymakers. The aim of this chapter is to discuss the role for science advisors to provide the main guarantee that the research, which provides the evidence for policymaking, is based on methodologically robust and ethically grounded scientific work. This relies on the academic training and culture of the science advisers. There is currently no forum where policymakers and academic/higher education institution (HEI) researchers can easily come together to work jointly to develop the process of continuous expert policy advice and evaluation in response to key national strategic issues. In progressing this agenda, it is critical to design effective structures to identify research demand from government and ethically sound research supply from HEIs and other sources over the long term, at least at national levels. Even more importantly, there are no declared standards in scientific policy advice, except the assumption that those who have received an academic training are assumed to be bounded by robust academic values and carry these with them into their new roles in providing scientific advice for policymaking. To explore this issue, this chapter examines the case of the International Network for Government Science Advice (INGSA). This is a gateway to the community of professional science advisers working inside governments, and to those engaged in other aspects of the production, brokerage and analysis of scientific advice, not just in the European Union (EU) but globally.

Keywords European Alliance for Social Sciences and Humanities (EASSH) · Evidence informed policy · Science advisor · International Network for Government Science Advice (INGSA)

G. Lombardo (✉)
European Alliance for Social Sciences and Humanities (EASSH), Paris, France
e-mail: gabi.lombardo@eassh.eu

© The Author(s) 2022
D. O'Mathúna and R. Iphofen (eds.), *Ethics, Integrity and Policymaking*, Research Ethics Forum 9, https://doi.org/10.1007/978-3-031-15746-2_6

67

6.1 Introduction

With around 6000 members from more than 100 countries, the International Network for Government Science Advice (INGSA) provides a forum for policymakers, practitioners, national academies, and academics to share experience, build capacity and develop theoretical and practical approaches to the use of scientific evidence in informing policy at all levels of government (for more information, see https://www. ingsa.org). INGSA is supported primarily by the Wellcome Trust and the International Development Research Centre. It operates under the auspices of the International Science Council and is managed through a secretariat based at the University of Auckland.

The INGSA case study provided here is an example of an existing, informal, network of key actors who play a role in building evidence and providing advice for the formation of public policy. INGSA membership is far wider than science advisors working in government ministries. It draws together a range of roles and experiences, which highlights an important fact of the contemporary dynamics behind policy advice and how the knowledge and policy production environment is changing fast. In a context of mission-oriented research and multi-stakeholder actors in knowledge creation, the evidence used to inform public opinion, civil servants and policies, and in general our society, is no longer generated just in academia and translated via a small number of controlled channels. Trusted sources of knowledge have traditionally been via academic publications in journals and monographs. In this knowledge society, evidence is generated in several different ways and translated through a plethora of new channels made up of think tanks, advisors, nongovernmental organisations (NGOs), and formal and informal infrastructures. The expression 'good evidence' can be limited and unclear. In fact, given the multiple pathways available to generate scientific evidence, what matters is being able to identify how transparent the process is and how straightforward the mechanism is to assess the liability of the evidence. This highlights the key role that science advisors play in this context to be able to source knowledge that has been constructed according to rigorous scientific methods and through research which has applied appropriate ethical standards.

The aim of this chapter tries to assess the science advisors' understandings and insights about the nature of the research they access to inform policymaking and how they establish that the feedback they communicate as evidence, originates from methodologically robust and ethically grounded research. Most of the literature on science advice is based on the capacity and the opportunity for experts to be able to "translate" science into policy and most importantly to be effective communicators, so that their advice has an impact on policymaking (Andrews 2017; Selin et al. 2017).

One of the important roles for a network like INGSA is to help prepare new scientific advisers. Many who take up these roles will have careers as full-time academics in universities and research institutes. The world of policymaking may remove them from their comfort zone. Policymaking moves quickly, and certainly more quickly than the conduct of most research. The modern scientific advisor may be asked to work beyond the boundaries of their scientific field, drawing together evidence for policymaking in complex multidimensional challenges, which require input from multiple disciplines. A network like INGSA can help to prepare scientists to work in very different ways to gather scientifically grounded evidence from across disciplines as evidence for policymaking.

INGSA provides such a platform for training and also to encourage the exchange of best practice between members of this community. At the core, INGSA has created an environment which recognises both international standards and is sensitive of geographical differences. Regular training is delivered to support academics who choose to become government advisors and to share understanding about how science advisors are trained and learn to identify scientific evidence which is fundamentally robust and ethically sound. The platform also supports critical training via case studies and real-life examples about the understanding of how science advisors must be aware of their own inherent biases and implicit political agendas that lie beyond the evidence and the research they access for policymaking advice.

It is not only those with the scientific backgrounds who benefit from training and the opportunity for discussions around best practice. The experts who advise policymakers could come from many different sectors and backgrounds. Several may be trained within government departments, civil servants, and policy organisations. Others emerge from the private sector, industry or NGOs and civil society stakeholders, professionals in different areas of knowledge. Another group emerges directly from scholarly research, generally working in academic institutions who may be invited to join expert groups and provide advisory functions after taking short-term roles and positions.

Over the last 10–15 years, and with a certain degree of 'acceleration' of influence that has happened more recently with the unprecedented COVID-19 pandemic, we have seen the emergence and proliferation of such mixed profiles. Science advisors have taken key places in supporting actors in legislative assemblies (such as the UK Parliament), shadowing Members of Parliament (MPs) to support their work with their portfolios, and advising officials with statutory powers (e.g., public bodies) when they are tasked with policy design and assessment.

Science advisors' profiles and their process of learning to become professionals have evolved rapidly, but as attention has mainly focused on how policymakers can access evidence for their work, less attention has been paid to how experts become advisors, or occasionally whether the advisors come from traditional 'expert' backgrounds (Owens 2015, 10). More importantly, attention has rarely been paid to how the advisors, particularly those with scientific backgrounds, are changed by the role they play in providing evidence for policymaking. It is unclear how they generate 'new knowledge' which is immediately translated in the realities of the political world. Many are required to undergo some transformation, as Obermeister (2020) says "they become 'policy literate'." In other words, they must move between the intricacies of political mechanisms and the generation of scientific evidence, while at the same time, they are also inevitably influenced by their own personal experiences, beliefs, values and cultural backgrounds (Spruijt et al. 2014; Porter and Dessai 2017). They may also witness instances of what they would consider 'policy-based evidence making' as opposed to evidence-based policymaking.

To further complicate the advising role, it has been observed that the relationship between science and policymaking has changed over time. According to Gluckman and Wilsdon (2016) science advice is an evolving (eco)system in which science advisors tend to constantly adapt. More importantly, this relationship has been made far more complex by the increasing capacity of different entities and organisations to provide evidence for policymaking. All advisors share some commonalities in the challenges they face, including: assuring independence and influence, preserving trust while becoming more transparent, and guaranteeing the quality of the advice they provide (Wilsdon 2014). Today, these ecosystems are more diverse than ever before and yet not quite as resilient as in previous decades.

6.2   Good Evidence and Transparency of Sources—Advisors or Science Advisors, and Does the Distinction Matter?

There is a tacit assumption that responsibility for the production of ethically robust research simply lies in the academic environment and that this assumption provides a level of assurance about the quality of the research itself. Although this is not disputed in principle, it may not be sufficient in a knowledge society and a research system which is now opening up, inviting a much wider range of collaborators working in the 'knowledge production space'. Some come with very different standards and approaches, and generate academic papers in collaboration with scholars. Without diminishing the importance of this approach, it assumes that all stakeholders share broadly similar fundamental assumptions, including beliefs about the validity of different knowledge sources, the importance of complexity, and the need to engage with the knowledge and values of relevant stakeholders.

What is missing is a framework which could sensitise organisations to evaluate the robustness of the environment in which evidence is generated. As part of the changes of the research system, the gradual inclusion of innovative knowledge generation mechanisms is occurring, particularly in addressing complex challenges and sustainable goals. We also must ensure that there are mechanisms which are widely used and coherently employed to assess any possible intrinsic bias in knowledge generation. As the vice-chair of INGSA and other practitioners in think tanks have underlined in the PRO-RES series of interviews (see PRO-RES deliverable D2.3 https://prores-project.eu/deliverables/), it is crucial to include tools for the assessment of scientific evidence wherever such evidence is generated, especially for research in non-medical science where there are less well established protocols for ethics.

A network like INGSA has a role to "establish protocols that are widely used and policymakers can take into account; have standards to identify when evidence is ethically robust; enforce protocols to discourage policymakers from using more 'convenient' evidence" James Wilsdon's interview (17 June 2020).

The above observation highlights an emerging new challenge for scientific advisors—an emerging marketplace of ideas. New actors play an increasingly important role in providing evidence to political policymakers who may find 'convenient evidence' provides a better justification for political policy development, which puts the role of the independent scientific adviser under increasing pressure. In the science-policy relationship there are competing actors, from journalists to think tanks, who play a very crucial role in informing societal changes, processes and procedures while claiming an evidence-based approach. They also generate new knowledge and evidence which are often more easily picked up by 'lay' (those not professional researchers) members of society who are in key decision-making roles.

These changes might suggest the need for wider exposure to the kind of training undertaken by academic researchers to identify the investigation underpinning evidence for policymaking which is ethically sound. However, as it is often discussed in academia, you cannot really propose some definitive standards or "do's and don'ts" when you are engaging with live social contexts and where the simple principle of "do no harm", for example, has a much larger spectrum of implications. See for example the ongoing discussion about technology and its role in society, or also as the COVID-19 pandemic has shown, how scientific advice has been employed to protect society's health and suppress negative impact on people's economic welfare or even their mental health. Science-advising for policymakers is not straightforward and cannot offer a pre-determined set of rules but must be based on long- and well-established practices, and flexible and adaptable platforms to identify transparent and ethically sound information, as well as exploiting formally trained and capable individuals with high standards of professional integrity.

6.3   Advising Governments: The International Network for Governmental Science Advisors (INGSA)

INGSA offers a collaborative platform which enables a valuable exchange among policymakers, scientists, and experts in key areas of knowledge at the international level. The platform also aims to support a certain level of capacity building and research networks across diverse global science advisory organisations and national systems. The platform mainly focuses on organising workshops, conferences and a growing catalogue of tools and guidance, which aims at improving the interface between global science-policy actors to enhance the potential for evidence-informed policy formation at sub-national, national and transnational levels. INGSA working groups are developed to take on targeted projects such as workshop planning and the development of publications and other resource materials (see e.g., https://www.ingsa.org/wp-content/uploads/2016/09/Swamperia.pdf).

INGSA's mission is to provide a forum for policymakers, practitioners, national academies, and academics to share experiences, build capacity and develop theoretical and practical approaches to the use of scientific evidence in informing policy at all levels of government. However, its primary focus is on the place of science in public policy formation rather than advice on the structure and governance of public science and innovation systems.

As their website (https://www.ingsa.org) claims, INGSA operates through:

- Exchanging lessons, evidence and new concepts through conferences, workshops and a website;
- Collaborating with other organisations with common or overlapping interests;
- Assisting the development of advisory systems through capacity-building workshops;
- Producing articles and discussion papers based on comparative research into the science and art of scientific advice.

In other words, INGSA is not trying to implement a framework within which science advice must be implemented but rather to create an open dialogue over the practices and the processes in use between different countries and cultures, and at the same time, to identify some overall principles for robust and effective results. INGSA's operational principles are based on a commitment to diversity and recognising and accepting multiple cultures and structures of governance and policy development. INGSA does not intend to lobby for, or endorse, any particular form or structure of science advice to governments. INGSA's primary objective is to improve the use of evidence in informing public policy, rather than providing advice on the structure and governance of public science and innovation systems.

Given the mission of an organisation like INGSA, it is recognised that the PRO-RES guidance framework (https://prores-project.eu), made of the Accord, the toolbox (https://prores-project.eu/toolbox-2/) and the resources (https://prores-project.eu/resources/) would be particularly important in supporting the training material developed by INGSA. The guidance framework is a collection of principles, values and standards for right action that is seen as morally binding upon the members of a group. The framework is designed to guide, control, and/or regulate proper and acceptable behaviour as it contains advice and guidance on how one 'ought' to behave in producing ethical evidence. More importantly, the toolbox offers a range of ways to operationalise the goals of the Accord and offers a 'how to' list for delivering ethical evidence.

Because of its nature, INGSA remains fundamentally a loosely-knit association of individuals and organisations with interests in both the theory and practice of science advice and it is based on a distributed operational model where members do not need to share the same physical location when interacting (see below). In the mind of INGSA's funders, it is expected that the network will be shaped and reshaped over time according to the arising needs and interests of INGSA affiliates. Such an approach fits very neatly in the ever-evolving nature of the PRO-RES framework which is based not on a rigid normative structure, as for example the Oviedo or Helsinki framework, but capitalises on the collection of case studies and experiences that ethics experts and literature on ethical approaches develop over time.

6.4   Feedback from INGSA

As mentioned above, INGSA is based on an informal, distributed operational model which delivers capacity building and convening through regional chapters. Such a model helps to contextualise the universal message and make it relevant locally. Operating through the global hub based in New Zealand, INGSA has three regional chapters in Latin America, Asia and Africa. This ensures better regional relevance, but also cross-regional and especially South-North/South-South collaboration and lesson sharing, which had previously been lacking at a global scale.

The interviews with senior representatives of INGSA revealed that a fundamental element of their work on science advice was about how to identify good evidence and describe what constitutes good evidence. Consideration of reputable science publications, high reputation scholars and research institutions, and reliable sources providing robust and reproducible results are crucial for identifying such good evidence—although they are sometimes not exhaustive and leave out a range of knowledge producers not coming from the top layer of the academic world but who could, nonetheless, contribute, particularly in niche research areas, or in areas of investigations very closely related to policymaking.

At the same time, senior representatives of INGSA recognised that ethically robust scientific evidence especially in non-medical sciences (including engineering, politics and finance for example) is far more difficult to identify 'downstream' when the research results have been translated and integrated into policy recommendations. Furthermore, the integrity of scholars in presenting their results is presumed, in part, to be guaranteed by the reputation of their host institution or the reputation of the scholars themselves. Yet, there are two related problems with such assumptions: firstly, does 'reputation' apply as a mark of quality to all the work undertaken by scholars in an institution or for each publication produced by an individual academic? In reality the quality of work underpinning 'reputation' will fall somewhere on a curve, with reputation in a research field based on a perceived mean created over decades. Peer review publications and other forms of academic engagement over a sustained period grant the due acknowledgement. However, this is no guarantee of work of consistent scientific quality across all research fields and peer review practices are sometimes criticised as considered non-standard practice (Smith 2006). The second is related to the proliferation of league tables produced by the higher education 'trade press'. These exercises are based on metrics selected according to what can be measured by the particular publication or publisher and not necessarily based on which metric provides a better insight into the quality of research underpinning a publication used as evidence for policymaking. Needless to say, whereas well developed and universal mechanisms exist to scrutinise and assess research results via peer review, when results are transformed into policy relevant 'evidence', especially where multiple studies are integrated and synthesised by non-academically trained contributors, little guidance exists to date to identify if the studies used were valid and reliable. Practical guidance is needed to assess whether reports have drawn on evidence according to high standards and formal guidance, or whether it has been collected for fast communication and dissemination. This is particularly challenging in certain research areas where such assessment is beyond the capacity of single advisors. This should not emerge as a surprise given that we are aware that ethics of research and integrity of scholars is increasingly implemented in scholars' training and that training in science advice has only emerged in recent years, not least through the efforts of INGSA.

As has been stated, INGSA does not provide evidence to policymakers directly. INGSA has the role of facilitator and promoter among academics to encourage them to engage in a career which includes advising policymakers, and among policymakers on seeking expert advice. Given this purpose for the organisation, INGSA focuses on encouraging those who advise policymakers to only use ethically robust evidence and more importantly to have a very high integrity of working methods especially in gathering and presenting information.

Finally, the INGSA distributed model confronts the difficulties that many platforms face. INGSA is a voluntary association of members and as such is a coordinated bottom-up effort to connect researchers with policymakers. It is also very sensitive of geographical and cultural differences, and preserves diversity of approaches and other multicultural and intellectual ventures. However, INGSA has not yet implemented a formal published declaration of the intentions, motives, or views which is recognised and endorsed by all members. Therefore, it still lacks a driving force which has enough authority across different constituencies to implement a set of projects fast enough to address the ever-changing relations between science and policy. Especially in the twenty-first century, international organisations seem to have a weakening position, whereas national governments have reasserted their sovereignty. The next step in INGSA's development will be to see how often researchers trained via INGSA's approaches will successfully engage and take positions as formal government advisors. At the moment, such positions remain strongly related to personal contacts and are subject to the changing of political parties in governments. Besides, we must bear in mind that part of the independence of researchers supporting policymakers is often guaranteed by their roles as advisors. Researchers and scientific advisors provide what they assess as the best possible scientific evidence, whereas the liability of the decision taken following such advice and sometimes multiple sources of advice, remains with the policymakers, the political appointees. INGSA is developing a strong platform and is a resource for strengthening evidence based policy, yet remains a fragile multifaceted platform.

6.5 Institutional Capacities: Improving Research Systems for Ethical Advice

In addition to building the capacity of individual researchers and policymakers to provide and request robust evidence, INGSA's work has an institutional layer regarding the integrity of the research ecosystem to allow the circulation of the best possible research evidence. Conversations with INGSA senior management have shown that their attention is focused on the importance of having in place a much stronger mechanism of incentives and rewards for those engaged in research and those that use research for their work. In fact, research ethics issues are often linked to moral choices. If we look at the debate around Open Science, reproducibility of data and assessments, all have some kind of normative frameworks, but it is not easy to just follow guidelines and instructions. For example, the FAIR (Findable Accessible Interoperable Re-Usable) principles could not simply be addressed from one single perspective (GO FAIR 2016). There are reasons why such principles emerge, and they do have an ethical dimension, but there are also other motives underlying research. In fact, the problem with the research system is that it does not offer enough incentives to hold ethics in high regard.

From INGSA's perspective, the core issue is the overall research system which starts with the researchers' training but moves along the complex picture of research methods, reward mechanisms and Open Science. Ethics is a keyhole to observe a much larger phenomenon around knowledge production. Those advocating for Open Science target the emergence of a fragmentation in knowledge production and science communicators who miss a strict academic training. Also, a strong trend towards open access publishing (OAP) of journals and books has encouraged the practice of peer-review post-publication as being a more transparent process. As many public funding agencies require OAP of results of funded research projects, publishers try to take advantage by offering OA platforms and a shift to article processing cost (APC) financing. Scientists themselves witness a rapidly changing landscape of established and recently emerging journals of mixed quality, ethics and aims.

TransDisciplinary Research (TDR) is the preferred pathway for mission-driven research and invites a multi-stakeholder engagement. The question is also how to assess TDR before, during and after the analysis. As mentioned in a very recent OECD paper "the science and policy communities need criteria to assess whether TDR proposals are likely to yield desired results, indicators to weigh the progress and sustainability of existing research efforts and ensure continued application of the principles of TD, and standards—practical, scientific, and ethical—for appraising the value of completed research" (OECD 2020, 16).

Although ethics remains a fundamental requirement for robust evidence, it is hard – and we could probably say—increasingly harder to assess robustness of the evidence generated and, more importantly, of any translation of such knowledge made available for the purpose of policymaking.

6.6 Science Advice in Emergencies—A Unique and Pressing Case for Ethics and Integrity

Beyond its training for individual scientists and policy professionals and its institutional advocacy to improve research systems, INGSA develops specific thematic projects from time to time. One such project is directly relevant to and complements the PRO-RES framework. In collaboration with its parent body, the International Science Council (ISC), INGSA has engaged in a project with ISC's Committee for Freedom and Responsibility in Science (https://council.science/about-us/govern ance/committees/committee-for-freedom-and-responsibility-in-science/) to support the development of specific guidance for expert advising in emergency and crisis situations.

In addition to adding a layer of urgency to the advice given, the speed and high stakes of crisis situations increases the potential for uncertainty and contestation of evidence. For this reason, applying an ethics- and integrity-based framework to the role of advising in emergencies is of critical importance. INGSA is engaged in thoroughly analysing the situation across multiple global regions, placing the organisation in an ideal position to ground the framework in local and crisis contexts.

6.7 Conclusions

The outcome of this INGSA case study demonstrates three main points:

(a) There is a proven market internationally, for learning the skills of robust and trustworthy knowledge brokerage, which INGSA's capacity building and convening activities have both responded to and have been working to develop further.
(b) INSGA's devolved model of program delivery and governance through regional chapters is key to putting issues of ethics and integrity into local context. At the same time, its work within the International Science Council and the Committee on Freedom and Responsibility of Scientists places these issues into the specific context of emergency and crisis situations.
(c) The PRO-RES framework is an important tool which can complement INGSA's work to help sensitise evidence-commissioning and provisioning organisations to work in ethically sound and methodologically robust ways.

At the same time the case study shows some weaknesses in the approach:

(a) The INGSA distributed model confronts the difficulties that many platforms face, with the lack of a driving force which has enough authority across different constituencies to implement a set of projects fast enough to address the ever-changing relations between science and policy.
(b) Understanding the implementation of ethically robust evidence cannot be based on a rigid normative framework with a simple list of rights and wrongs, but the advice must be adjusted to the diversity of culture and society, to the rapidly changing dynamics of scientific discoveries and endless policy demands which emerge at very different speeds with various implications for time lags.

Apart from INGSA, there are some more recent national and international mechanisms seeking to fill this space. This means that together with the fragmentation of knowledge producers we may soon have to face the proliferation of standards for knowledge translators and advisors who find the ears of policymakers. In reality, this is already the case.

References

Andrews, L. 2017. How can we demonstrate the public value of evidence-based policy making when government ministers declare that the people 'have had enough of experts'? *Palgrave Communications* 3: 11. https://doi.org/10.1057/s41599-017-0013-4.

Beddington, J. 2013. The science and art of effective advice. In *Future Directions for Scientific Advice in Whitehall*, ed. R. Doubleday and J. Wilsdon, 22–31. Cambridge: Centre for Science and Policy.

Bijker, W.E., R. Bal, and R. Hendriks R. 2009. *The Paradox of Scientific Authority: The Role of Scientific Advice in Democracies*. Cambridge: MIT Press.

DTL (Digital Life Science). 2016. European Commission embraces the FAIR principles. Dutch Techcentre for Life Sciences. https://www.dtls.nl/2016/04/20/european-commission-allocates-e2-billion-to-make-research-data-fair. Accessed 2 January 2022.

GO FAIR. 2016. FAIR principles. https://www.go-fair.org/fair-principles/. Accessed 2 January 2022.

Gluckman, P., and J. Wilsdon. 2016. From paradox to principles: Where next for scientific advice to governments? *Palgrave Communications* 2: 16077. https://doi.org/10.1057/palcomms.2016.77.

Moore, A.J. 2017. *Critical Elitism: Deliberation, Democracy, and the Problem of Expertise*. New York: Cambridge University Press.

Obermeister, N. 2020. Tapping into science advisers' learning. *Palgrave Communications* 6: 74. https://doi.org/10.1057/s41599-020-0462-z.

OECD. 2020. Addressing societal challenges using transdisciplinary research. OECD Science, Technology and Industry Policy Papers, No. 88. Paris: OECD Publishing. https://doi.org/10.1787/0ca0ca45-en.

Owens, S. 2015. *Knowledge, Policy, and Expertise: The UK Royal Commission on Environmental Pollution 1970–2011*. New York: Oxford University.

Porter, J.J., and S. Dessai. 2017. Mini-me: Why do climate scientists' misunderstand users and their needs? *Environmental Science & Policy* 77: 9–14. https://doi.org/10.1016/j.envsci.2017.07.004.

Selin, N.E., L.C. Stokes, and L.E. Susskind. 2017. The need to build policy literacy into climate science education. *WIRES Climate Change* 8: e455. https://doi.org/10.1002/Wcc.455.

Smith, R. 2006. Peer review: A flawed process at the heart of science and journals. *Journal of the Royal Society of Medicine* 99: 178–182.

Spruijt, P., A.B. Knol, E. Vasileiadou, J. Devilee, E. Lebret, and A.C. Petersen. 2014. Roles of scientists as policy advisers on complex issues: a literature review. *Environmental Science and Policy* 40: 16–25. https://doi.org/10.1016/j.envsci.2014.03.002.

Wilsdon, J. 2014. The past, present and future of the Chief Scientific Advisor. *European Journal of Risk and Regulations* 5: 293–299. https://doi.org/10.1017/S1867299X00003809.

Chapter 7
The PRO-RES Guidance Framework for Scientific Research: A Novel Response to Long-Standing Issues

P. Kavouras and C. A. Charitidis

Abstract For more than three quarters of a century the large-scale application of superconductors demanded the use of expensive liquid helium, rendering large-scale application of superconductors unfeasible. The only way out of this deadlock was the invention of high temperature or high T_C superconductors. In 1986, J.G. Bednorz and K.A. Müller demonstrated superconductivity at the record temperature of 30 K. This publication fostered a scientific research rush that culminated in the development, by P. Chu, of a material that turned into a superconductor below 93 K. The stakes could not be higher from academic, technological and economic perspectives, since high T_C superconductivity could bring a Nobel Prize in Physics to its creators, would open up the way to commercial applications of superconductors, triggering a major technological revolution, and most possibly, create a multibillion-dollar market. In this chapter, we discuss cases of possible breaches of research integrity that occurred during the so-called "race for the superconductor", as was chronicled in the book "The Breakthrough: The Race for the Superconductor" by R.M. Hazen, vis-à-vis the values and principles established within the PRO-RES normative framework, which is being built to merge the principles of Responsible Research and Innovation (RRI), required from researchers, and research funding and performing organizations, with an aim to balance political, institutional and professional contradictions and constraints.

Keywords Research ethics · Research integrity · Misconduct · PRO-RES project · Guidance framework · Informed policy decision

7.1 Introduction

Superconductors were discovered by the Dutch physicist Heike Kamerlingh Onnes in 1911, in Leiden, in The Netherlands (van Delft 2007). A superconductor is a material that possesses zero electrical resistance and completely expulses magnetic fields below a specific temperature that is called the critical temperature of T_C (Ashcroft

P. Kavouras (✉) · C. A. Charitidis
School of Chemical Engineering, National Technical University of Athens, Athens, Greece
e-mail: kavouras@chemeng.ntua.gr

© The Author(s) 2022
D. O'Mathúna and R. Iphofen (eds.), *Ethics, Integrity and Policymaking*, Research Ethics Forum 9, https://doi.org/10.1007/978-3-031-15746-2_7

and Mermin 1976). Even though such physical properties are definitely extremely useful for a myriad of applications, they occur in temperatures near absolute zero, i.e. 0 K or -273.15 °C. This posed an insurmountable barrier for the application of superconductors at the time of their discovery. For more than three quarters of a century the T_C for the appearance of superconductivity increased from 4.2 to 23 K, reflecting a rather hectic progress. As a result, superconducting devices needed to be cooled down with the use of expensive liquid helium, rendering any large-scale application of superconductors unfeasible. The only way out of this deadlock was the invention of high T_C superconductors, meaning the production of superconducting materials with T_C higher than liquid nitrogen temperature (i.e., $T_C \geq 77$ K), since liquid nitrogen is about 100 times cheaper than liquid helium. High T_C superconductors had been turned into a chimera, while the related scientific research was sometimes described (not always with the best of intentions) as the quest for the "Holy Grail" of materials science or "modern Alchemy".

Stagnant waters were stirred in 1986, when two IBM scientists working in Zurich, Switzerland, Johann Georg Bednorz and Karl Alex Müller demonstrated superconductivity in a metal oxide well above the previous temperature threshold. Their publication did not cause great excitement. The scientific literature abounded with publications announcing alleged high T_C superconductors, only to be withdrawn after the first failed replication tests. The superconductor scientific community was fatigued and disappointed, showing signs of indifference. However, physicist Paul Chu from the University of Houston, USA, based on Bednorz and Müller, developed a completely new material that became a superconductor below 93 K, well above the temperature of cheap liquid nitrogen! This invention could trigger a technological revolution, a breakthrough of monumental magnitude, since it rendered commercial applications of superconductors feasible.

The stakes were extremely high; at the beginning of 1987 Chu was a potential Nobel laureate in Physics and his Institute (the University of Houston) could benefit (as long as the right patenting strategy was followed) from an invention that was bound to create a multibillion-dollar market. In a completely different tone, the story of the revolutionary invention of high T_C superconductors reveals possible breaches of research integrity, and raises questions about whether misconduct, like falsification of research results, or questionable research practices, like partitioning a large study that could have been reported in a single research article into smaller published articles (salami slicing), might have occurred.

Nowadays, having the prior experience of the discussions related to the "reproducibility crisis" the above unsettling issues might not seem to be "in a completely different tone". Beginning with the publication by John Ioannidis who claimed in 2005 that "*most published research findings are false*" (Ioannidis 2005), numerous statistical surveys (Baker 2016), meta-research articles (Bohannon 2015; Iqbal et al. 2016) and replication studies (Baker and Dolgin 2017) have been published, especially during the last decade, showing that a significant output of scientific research cannot be reproduced or replicated. While Ioannidis' publication exposed methodological shortcomings in current research, like the use of insufficient empirical data and poor use of statistical methods, it also brought about issues related to the research environment, such as the pressure to publish, as causes of scientific results' irre-producibility. Since the early 2010s discussions about these issues have been in full fledge, during which a constellation of additional causes of non-reproducible results have been brought to light, like flawed calibration or improper accreditation of measuring instruments, lack of Standard Operating Procedures (SOPs), and poor mentorship.

The authors wish to declare that they have made the analysis presented in this chapter based on the information published in Robert M. Hazen's, *The Breakthrough: The Race for the Superconductor* (1988). The authors used the Greek translation of this book, published under the title "Η ΡΗΞΗ—Η κούρσα της υπεραγωγιμότητας" by ΤΡΟΧΑΛΙΑ editions (1990) ISBN: 960–7022-11-4 (Hazen 1990). This case study is presented in six sections reflecting a periodization that follows the different phases the research for the superconductor went through. These phases expose different types of ethical dilemmas and/or types of possible breaches of research integrity, as well as interaction with different types of stakeholders. A rough timeline of the case study is schematically presented in Fig. 7.1. In these six sections, we present cases of possible data manipulation, appli-cation of questionable research practices, sloppy science, and attempts to manipulate researchers either by policy makers (based on arguments of national security) or by research administrators (based on arguments of economic benefits).

After the end of each section, we make a connection to the most relevant content of the PRO RES project normative guidance framework. This connection has been structured following the different types of resources found at the project's website. More specifically, the reader will find:

- A list of questions that help the reader reflect on the decisions and actions of the researchers and other stakeholders involved in the "race for the superconductor".
- A collection of the relevant terms from the PRO-RES glossary. These terms refer to the principles at stake or describe potential types of misconduct that emerge from the content of each section.
- Comments, based on the PRO-RES framework; more specifically from: (a) the foundational statements for ethical research practice and (b) the supporting Toolbox.

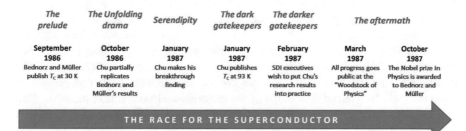

The prelude	The Unfolding drama	Serendipity	The dark gatekeepers	The darker gatekeepers	The aftermath	
September 1986	October 1986	January 1987	January 1987	February 1987	March 1987	October 1987
Bednorz and Müller publish T_c at 30 K	Chu partially replicates Bednorz and Müller's results	Chu makes his breakthrough finding	Chu publishes T_c at 93 K	SDI executives wish to put Chu's research results into practice	All progress goes public at the "Woodstock of Physics"	The Nobel prize in Physics is awarded to Bednorz and Müller

THE RACE FOR THE SUPERCONDUCTOR

Fig. 7.1 Schematic diagram of a rough timeline of the "race for the superconductor" and this chapter's sections

This chapter concludes with an overall exposition of the basic problematic posed during the "race for the superconductor". The authors drafted this section with the aid of another element of the PRO-RES framework, namely the "Accord", which is the focal point of the PRO-RES framework, bringing together all the other constitutive elements of the framework with a set of succinct, high-level statements.

7.2   The Prelude

Bednorz and Müller, based on the findings of Claude Michel from the University of Caen, France, who had produced copper oxide-based compounds with surprisingly high conductivity, succeeded in revealing superconductivity with the very same compounds at the record T_C of 30 K. Despite the fact that this result was confirmed beyond any doubt on January 1986, the two researchers submitted the related manuscript three months later in the not so famous journal *Zeitschrift Für Physik* (Bednorz and Müller 1986). The two researchers had some relations with the editorial team that ensured a degree of confidentiality during the reviewing process, as described by Hazen (1990). Even after the manuscript was accepted for publication the two researchers kept a low profile and they did not reveal their discovery, not even to their colleagues in IBM. Their article was published in September 1986, without causing any kind of scientific elation whatsoever.

This paper was taken seriously by physicist Paul Chu from the University of Houston, USA. Chu was struggling to get funding for his research on superconductivity, an endeavour that was becoming more and more difficult, since high T_C superconductivity was stubbornly resisting appearance, despite the efforts of two generations of scientists. Chu and his team saw the publication of Bednorz and Müller as a *Deus Ex Machina* revealing its presence from the other side of the Atlantic. They seized the opportunity; and they seized it "big time".

Chu and his team began studying this new material by making a replication study, i.e. a study to synthesize the material from scratch and confirm the alleged superconductivity at $T_C = 30$ K. The experimental protocol for replicating the research in superconductivity was to: (a) synthesize the alleged superconducting compound, (b) track T_C, (c) reveal the existence of the "Meissner effect" and (d) isolate and characterize the crystallographic structure of the superconducting phase, since the superconducting compound of Bednorz and Müller would, most probably, be composed of several different materials. Chu and his team succeeded in reproducing superconductivity at 30 K, but they were sceptical to announce such a result to a scientific community that was indifferent to such "Messianic" findings. After all, they had followed only two out of four steps of the experimental verification protocol. Chu and his team continued to work day and night following a laborious process of trial and error, until something happened: on the 25th of November 1986 their experimental devices showed superconductive transition at 73 K!

7.2.1   List of Questions

- Why did Bednorz and Müller follow a low profile during the publication process of their research?
- Was the replication study of Chu complete, considering that he had not followed the experimental protocol for recognizing superconductivity?

7.2.2   Relevant Terms from the PRO-RES Glossary

Accountability, Collaboration, Confidentiality, Honesty, Reliability.

7.2.3   Comments

Bednorz and Müller submitted their research to a peer reviewed journal which the two researchers had some connection with the editorial team thus ensuring a degree of confidentiality during the review process. We cannot assume that these relationships would necessarily serve the cause of a lenient review procedure, since the authors were accountable and their results were reliable as history proved. Also, we cannot assume that they were seeking a swift review procedure, since they were not acting under pressure; at the time they submitted their milestone paper research on high T_C superconductors was stagnant. If they wished for a swift publication, they would have submitted to another journal. If we assume that their choice was made for the sake of confidentiality, i.e. that the review of their manuscript would not be intentionally delayed, in order for their results to be copied by another research group, and their success denied, we can speculate that they might be sceptical of the honesty of the reviewers of other, perhaps more illustrious scientific journals.

One might agree that they knew that it was a significant contribution to the field of high T_C superconductors that deserved publication in a journal that would guarantee the highest possible impact. So, the authors faced a dilemma over which journal to submit their work to. Should they submit to a journal with guaranteed confidentiality during the review process and questionable impact, or to a journal with guaranteed impact and perhaps questionable confidentiality in the review process? In other words, the two researchers had to select between the options of either safeguarding their potential professional success or safeguarding the impact of their work. Bednorz and Müller opted for the first choice.

This brings forward an ethical dilemma that a researcher may have to confront during her/his professional life. Both concerns, as described above, are totally legitimate, i.e. demand recognition for one's work and strive for a high scientific/societal impact; however, they have a different quality. The former is related to the benefit of the two researchers, while the latter is related to the benefit of science and society at large. Certainly, *Zeitschrift Für Physik* cannot be considered a "rogue" publication, meaning that the results of Bednorz and Müller's research would have found their way to the scientific community sooner or later. In any case, Bednorz and Müller's choice, as proved by the course of events, did not delay research into high T_C superconductivity.

On the other side of the Atlantic, and in contrast to his European colleagues, Chu was acting under pressure, since he was struggling to secure funding for his research group. It his case we see that he was convinced from the findings of Bednorz and Müller, since he and his group put a lot of effort into the perovskite system that showed superconductivity at 30 K, even though they did not apply the complete replication protocol. The fact that Chu refrained from publishing a replication study cannot be based, at this point, on a desire to keep his findings secret or on a lack of collaborative spirit but rather as a sign of accountability. His group had not applied the replication protocol in its entirety, so a replication study would not have sufficient data to certify Bednorz and Müller's findings. One might even argue that he had the intuition that something important could be hiding behind this perovskite system that he wished to study in depth before going public.

7.2.4 Connection to the PRO-RES Toolbox

This section is mostly related to the PRO-RES toolbox via the "*WHEN and WHERE was the research/analysis conducted?*" queries. Other queries taken from the PRO-RES toolbox may be also relevant, to a lesser degree. This query set the scene for the quest from Chu's research group and defines, to a certain degree, the ethical issues that appeared as the story proceeded, according to Hazen (1990). The context within which the research was carried out was the one of a small research group that was facing existential problems, since future funding was by no means guaranteed. The research site was a University that it had to compete with other research performing organisations with significantly larger resources and more personnel. This setting gave Chu's group a serious handicap regarding research performance; it rendered adherence to research integrity more challenging.

7.3 The Unfolding Drama

Chu knew that to make quicker progress, he had to consult an expert in X-Ray Diffraction (XRD) analysis; he had to structurally characterize his "super" samples. Also, he would not go to a state-of-the-art laboratory since his finding would most likely not be kept secret. Chu might expect that once such a breakthrough discovery was revealed, industrial laboratories like those of AT&T Bell Labs, Westinghouse, or IBM Research would start devoting their excellent manpower and vast resources to study his samples, not to mention prestigious academic opponents like Stanford,

Berkeley or Northwestern Universities or Argonne National Laboratory. Chu would have been outrun and his path to glory would have been lost forever. This may be why he chose the XRD laboratory of Simon Moss (a renowned expert in XRD analysis) that was almost next door. Moss provided one of the PhD candidates he supervised to help Chu with the crystallographic analysis of the alleged high T_C superconductor.

What Chu did not know was that during December 1986 a "gold rush" for high T_C superconductors was in full swing. While Chu's group was making serious progress breaking one T_C record after another, without announcing anything, on 27 December 1986 a Beijing newspaper announced that Chinese scientists had discovered a compound that became a superconductor at 70 K; however, this article was shown to be inaccurate after a few months. According to Hazen (1990), Chu's research group started working under a cloud of mutual suspicion, since Chu believed that he had an informer in his team as most were of Chinese origin. At this point the whole research fervour went public. The *New York Times* published a front-page article on 30 December 1986. Even though the article mistakenly gave the lead in the research to Bell Labs, it raised public awareness of the incipient breakthrough in the field of superconductors.

Chu realized that he was about to lose the advantage of being the first to announce high T_C superconductivity. He announced his replication of Bednorz and Müller's discovery to the Annual Congress of Materials Research at the beginning of 1987. His presentation was interrupted by Koichi Kitazawa, a Japanese professor of industrial chemistry from the University of Tokyo, who was possibly forced to announce that the superconducting phase of Bednorz and Müller was isolated and almost fully characterized by his team. The key to the discovery of higher T_C superconductors lay in the hands of the Japanese and it would only be a matter of time before they discovered the "super" samples Chu's group had produced a few weeks previously. To complicate things, the replication of Bednorz and Müller's results from Houston and Tokyo Universities produced a cascade effect: almost immediately, dozens of laboratories all over the world started studying the superconductivity of the La–Ba–Cu–O system. For Chu it was time to publish; he hastily prepared a manuscript entitled: "Evidence for *superconductivity above 40 K* in the La-Ba-Cu–O compound system" in *Physical Review Letters (PRL)*, which was eventually published on 26 January 1987 and *since has received more than 1800 citations* (Chu et al. 1987a). Four days later another paper by Chu was published in the journal *Science* entitled: "Superconductivity at 52.5 K in the lanthanum-barium-copper-oxide system" which has *received almost 300 citations* (Chu et al. 1987b).

7.3.1   List of Questions

- Do you find Chu's decision to avoid going to a state-of-the-art laboratory a wise one?
- Do you think that Chu should not have made the announcement at the Annual Congress of Materials Research?

- Do you think that Chu was following "salami slicing" for his papers?
- If yes, why do you think he followed this path?

7.3.2   Terms from the PRO-RES Glossary

Accountability, Collaboration, Conflict of interest, Confidentiality, Cooperation, Misrepresentation, Publication ethics, Questionable Research Practices, Reliability, Transparency, Vested interests.

7.3.3   Comments

According to Hazen (1990), Chu was reluctant to send his samples to a state-of-the-art laboratory. Chu evidently believed that giving his samples to Moss ran a lower risk of exposing his valuable findings. Someone might think that this reflects a lack of collaborative spirit in Chu. However, it is difficult to believe that Chu made up his mind to go for Moss only based on a "perverse" gut feeling. Perhaps there were rumours or instances when state-of-the-art laboratories had broken research confidentiality. In any case, even if Chu's decision was not based on such a suspicion, Moss' laboratory and his excellent scientific record guaranteed that the structural characterization would be of the highest quality, despite not being conducted with the most sophisticated instruments.

Even though Chu kept secret his latest findings, he was forced to reveal the replication of Bednorz and Müller's findings to the Annual Congress of Materials Research. He made this decision despite the fact that he had not applied the full replication protocol. Chu had neither isolated nor characterized the crystallographic structure of the superconducting phase that was still waiting to reveal its secrets at Moss' laboratory. Is it a case of questionable research practice or lack of accountability and reliability? If Chu had mentioned that only two of the four steps of the replication protocol had been applied, i.e. if he had been transparent, would he have followed a more accurate communication path?

What, perhaps, is more interesting and challenging is the reason why he made such an announcement. If he just wanted to spread the word about the research he was doing, then he should also reveal his latest finding. But this was not the case; it seems that he aimed at putting his name and his laboratory on the list of those that, at that time, were at the forefront of high T_C superconductivity research, by disclosing the most "innocent" information. Was there an issue of misrepresentation or lack of collaborative spirit? Under the circumstances in which Chu was acting it might have been unfair for him to answer the above question affirmatively. Most probably other scientists kept secret their progress in order to retain a strategic advantage; e.g. Professor Kitazawa actually interrupted Chu to announce that his laboratory had already applied three out of the four replication steps, most probably to also declare that his group was also at the forefront of the quest for high T_C superconductivity. Chu was either brave enough or too hasty to be the first to "break the silence" among the research community. This resulted in others stepping up to make their appearance into what later culminated as the "race for the superconductor".

When Chu published two articles that announced T_C above 40 K, he already had indications for even higher T_C, according to Hazen (1990). Someone could argue that Chu just published what he was absolutely sure of. Someone else might argue that he was salami slicing his work. Considering the above discussion, which exposes the heavy conflict of interest between the research groups that were examining Bednorz and Müller's work, Chu's decision can be seen as a delicate balance between getting credit for increasing T_C from 30 K to 40 or 52.5 K, while not exposing his even more exciting findings, assuming those were too recent and not yet verified.

Perhaps the most challenging situation for Chu and his research group was that their work environment had become toxic. After the publication in a Chinese newspaper of an alleged breakthrough, Chu worried that he had an informer in his group releasing information on the ongoing experiments; i.e. he feared being the victim of "research espionage". This worry was deepening since most of Chu's co-workers were of Chinese origin. Considering that research needs a completely open exchange of information, at least between co-workers putting the pieces of information together, such suspicions could have delayed if not completely halted Chu's research. We do not know whether Chu discussed this with his co-workers, but we believe this fear put an extra burden in a challenging situation, i.e. when the research group needed to work almost non-stop to catch their real or imagined rivals.

7.3.4   Connection to the PRO-RES Toolbox

This section mostly relates to the PRO-RES toolbox question: "*HOW was the research/data-gathering and analysis conducted?*" An overarching issue here is the transparency of those conducting the research, and their offering clear justifications/rationale for the methods used. The details were provided above of the original protocol to replicate a study that was widely known and accepted. Chu's team deviated from this, according to Hazen (1990), since they had achieved synthesizing a material with the same T_C but their continuing endeavours were based on a partially applied replication protocol. As a result, the robustness of their future experiments could be questioned by someone without the prior knowledge of their eventual success. We might see here evidence of bias from Chu's side: having partly replicated Bednorz and Müller's findings he fully accepted the possibility of achieving higher T_C at the same system. This apparently risky decision emanates from the pressure Chu was experiencing in keeping his research group funded and given his limited resources at that time. The fact that he succeeded does not weaken the argument that his decision was not fully evidence-based.

7.4   Serendipity

Chu's submission to *PRL* was accepted, but Christmas holidays intervened and its publication was delayed for two weeks. In the meantime, the administration of the University of Houston realized that something with potentially significant economic benefit was coming into being at Chu's laboratory. Chu was convinced by his university's administration to submit for a patent, before his article appeared in *PRL*. The patent was submitted on 12 December 1986.

However, all these events did not really matter; Chu was on the verge of making the discovery of his life. By combining results indicating that T_C was increasing with increased pressure and pure intuition, having to do with vague structural considerations (please keep in ming that the crystallography of Chu's La-Ba-Cu–O was mostly unknown), Chu and his research team produced a superconductor with a T_C close to 100 K! That meant that cheap liquid nitrogen could be used, instead of expensive liquid helium, to transform *this* material into a superconductor. This was a discovery with potential momentous implications. A really high T_C superconductor could create a multibillion-dollar market and could lead to applications with beneficial societal impact. *This* material, created on 29 January 1987, did not contain lanthanum but yttrium instead; the "miracle" material was based on the Y–Ba–Cu–O system.

The time to apply the full experimental protocol had come: Chu had to make the delicate measurement for the occurrence of the Meissner Effect, so he sent the precious samples to Chao-Yuan Huang of Los Alamos laboratories in New Mexico. He also had to isolate and fully characterize the structure of the superconductive phase. Then problems started. At the beginning, for the sake of confidentiality, Chu tasked one of his co-workers to characterize the superconductive phase; that proved to be a tantalizing undertaking, since this co-worker did not have substantial experience in XRD analysis. Chu again had to trust Moss's experimental equipment, but Chu did NOT reveal the exact composition to Moss, again according to Hazen (1990). As soon as the preliminary analysis was concluded, Chu pushed Moss to publish. Both men seemed to realize that the stakes were extremely high. However, their approach was fundamentally different. Moss refused to publish until a complete crystallographic analysis was made; that meant clarifying the composition and exact stoichiometry of the "miracle" sample. Chu refused and his cooperation with Moss came to an abrupt end.

7.4.1   List of Questions

- What should be the guiding principle when a scientist must decide whether there is a need to protect a discovery by a patent, before openly announcing her/his findings?
- Was Moss' refusal to cooperate with Chu justifiable?

7.4.2   Terms from the PRO-RES Glossary

Collaboration, Conflict of interest, Confidentiality, Cooperation, Questionable Research Practices, Reliability, Transparency.

7.4.3   Comments

Chu seems to have been uninterested in patenting the superconducting materials he and his group had synthesized at the end of 1986. This might be because high T_C superconductivity would have really mattered, in technological terms, only if T_C would have superseded liquid nitrogen temperature. Chu might not have had time to think about commercial exploitation of his findings. It is true, however, that when the University's lawyer suggested a patent, Chu submitted one before his article on a T_C at 40 K was published, despite knowing that this finding was already outpaced by his own work. This is an instance where a researcher should decide either to communicate her/his findings unconditionally openly or try to protect them via a patent—meaning that communication would have to be postponed altogether until the acceptance of the patent. This decision must be made by answering a question that leads to another dilemma: What are the responsibilities of a researcher working on a publicly funded research project? If the answer is "the promotion of knowledge and increased societal welfare", then a peer reviewed publication or an announcement at a scientific conference should be the first step in a chain of communication activities. If the answer is "commercialization of the research results and profit making", then a peer reviewed publication or any other kind of open communication has to wait.

This question is not so straightforward since the decision involves other stake-holders as well. In this case, the patent suggestion came from a lawyer working for the University of Houston, i.e. Chu's employer. A whole spectrum of new questions arises: Was Chu coerced to submit for a patent? Do the interests of a researcher and her/his employer coincide? Should they coincide? If they do not coincide, is there a danger of creating conflicts of interest? Did Chu refrain from patenting just to accelerate the publication of his findings? Is this an ethical reason to opt out of patenting? Should we leave the decision to the researcher or to the University administration?

Chu, after realizing that his methodology had produced superconductivity above liquid nitrogen temperature, decided to apply the complete characterization protocol. With that decision, necessary for his invention to be accepted for publication and for his group to receive credit, he again had to ensure there were no "leaks" from his collaborating laboratories. However, this time the stakes were much higher than a few months before. This led to a dramatic change in Chu's collaborative spirit that clashed with his undisputed excellence as a researcher. Fearing that Moss might disclose the composition of his "miracle" samples to rivals, Chu refused to reveal their exact composition—a practice that delayed Moss' study. Later, when Moss insisted that more experiments were needed to have a complete crystallographic characterization, Chu was pushing to publish without delay.

We see here an evident lack of cooperation and transparency from Chu's side. In addition, Chu's refusal to disclose the exact composition was directly affecting the speed and reliability with which the crystallographic analysis could be applied. Chu had involved Moss in a vicious circle, where Chu was willing to compromise the reliability of the crystallographic analysis, while being unwilling to compromise the safety of his findings. However, this conundrum can also be seen from a different perspective: Chu was focused on the "*how*" to synthesize the "miracle" superconductor, while Moss was focused on "*why*" this was a miracle superconductor, since crystallography could give greater insight into the physical mechanisms responsible for high T_C superconductivity. Moss escaped from this vicious circle by nullifying its cause: the cooperation with Chu.

7.4.4   Connection to the PRO-RES Toolbox

This section is mostly related to the PRO-RES toolbox question "*WHY was the research/enquiry/analysis conducted?*" The research was conducted to synthesize a superconductor with a T_C higher than that of liquid nitrogen. Chu was pushing the pace of his research group effort, despite that fact that they had already beaten Bednorz and Müller's achievement. Since the research began as soon as Bednorz and Müller's publication appeared, we can assume that there was no funding specifically for this effort to attain even higher T_C. So, Chu was not obliged to report his group's findings at any stage of the research. This brings forth the possibility that Chu had to pause all the other research being conducted by his group in order to deploy all available resources and manpower to achieve his ambition. This might, as well, have put extra pressure on him and his team.

7.5   The Dark Gatekeepers

Chu started writing a manuscript entitled "Superconductivity at 93 K in a new mixed-phase Y–Ba–Cu–O compound system at ambient pressure" for submission to *PRL*. He was aware that the two experts assigned to review the manuscript would be, most possibly, his scientific competitors. Even though they were bound by a confidentiality agreement, Chu was suspicious that they would try to take advantage, since they would have access to cutting edge information. Chu tried to convince *PRL*'s chief editor, to publish his manuscript **without** going through the peer review process; his request was turned down. Chu, then, suggested putting asterisks at the place of the chemical composition of his "miracle" material; the chief editor refused again. The two men agreed on the following path of the reviewing process, due to the extraordinary significance of the manuscript: according to Hazen (1990) the reviewers were selected by both Chu and the chief editor and their names would remain undisclosed to everyone else. The manuscript was submitted on 6 February 1987 and, in just 4 days, was accepted for publication.

A triumph of research integrity? Let's not jump to conclusions yet. Chu's manuscript contained two inaccuracies:

i. Instead of yttrium (Y) the manuscript contained ytterbium (Yb)[1] in the elemental composition.
ii. Instead of $Y_{1.2}Ba_{0.8}CuO_4$ the manuscript contained another stoichiometry, the mistaken formula: $Yb_{1.2}Ba_{0.8}CuO$.

Right after the submission of the manuscript, rumours of a new Yb-based superconductor had spread among the scientific community studying superconductivity. The news had leaked. On 18 February 1987, a week AFTER his manuscript was accepted, Chu sent the corrections on the elemental composition and the stoichiometry. The article was published on 2 March 1987 and shook the superconductor community; _since then it has received more than 9000 citations_ (Wu et al. 1987).

7.5.1 List of Questions

- What were Chu's incentives, if we assume that he intentionally changed the formula?
- Do you think that Chu knew that the Yb compound or the mistaken stoichiometry was not producing a superconductor? Does it make any difference?
- Were researchers that tested Yb justified in accusing Chu of data manipulation?
- Should the scientists that "confirmed" Yb superconductivity be held responsible for scientific misconduct?
- Should *PRL* be held responsible for the leaks?

7.5.2 Terms from the PRO-RES Glossary

Conflict of interest, Confidentiality, Deceit, Editorial misconduct, Falsification, Fraud, Publication ethics, Reliability, Research misconduct, Transparency.

---

[1] An interesting twist of fate is that Yb-based compounds did actually reveal superconductivity! Universities of Tokyo and Tohoku (Japan), as well as IBM and Bell Laboratories (USA), at the beginning of March 1987 "confirmed" the initially manipulated and unpublished manuscript of Chu.

7.5.3 Comments

Since the inception of peer review all publications deemed to be of scientific value and bearing a minimum of accountability must be reviewed by at least two experienced researchers, ideally from the same field of research. Reviewing is blind, meaning that the author(s) do not know the identity of the reviewers. Chu, breaking this tradition, suggested to the chief editor of *PRL*, a highly respected journal, to publish his manuscript without peer review. We cannot know if Chu really anticipated that the chief editor would take such a suggestion seriously. In any case, Chu succeeded in convincing him to apply the review process, but not a blind one. We leave it up to the readers to comment whether such a seemingly modest concession on the chief editor's part is justifiable. Did it increase transparency? One might assume that if the chief editor was absolutely certain of the confidentiality of *PRL*'s reviewers he would not have any reason to agree to such a procedure. Perhaps Chu had made clear that if such a concession had not been made, he would seek another journal to publish his revolutionary results. So, the chief editor would lose the opportunity to have in his journal a publication that had the potential to be the work of the decade. A small concession in publication procedures could increase *PRL*'s impact factor significantly.

The last argument might become more convincing after the last-minute corrections Chu made in the manuscript. These corrections were not just some details of the experimental protocol; they were substantial changes that, one could argue, should have caused a second round of review or even a re-submission. On the contrary, the corrections appeared in the *PRL* article without any repercussions whatsoever. However, the crucial discussion is about whether Chu intentionally manipulated the composition and stoichiometry of his miracle superconductors in the original manuscript, i.e. whether Chu had done research misconduct by manipulating his results. Considering that Chu was a renowned expert in the semiconductor community and the magnitude of his invention, it is very difficult to assume that he could have made such a mistake that, in addition, his collaborators had not noticed. On the other hand, Chu did not actually publish the allegedly manipulated results; he just put the symbol of a different element in the place of Y at the manuscript, instead of putting an asterisk as he had requested in the first place prior to the review. Since we cannot draw a definitive conclusion, we leave this cardinal question to our readers' judgment.

Deceitful or careless, overstretched by strenuous work or just sloppy, Chu's invention would have lost its lustre if he had followed *PRL*'s review procedure to the letter. Some might argue that if Chu manipulated his original manuscript then he did commit research misconduct. However, things in life are not always black and white; Chu was correct to doubt the confidentiality of the review process. Chu knew very well that the existing conflicts of interest with his rivals had skyrocketed. So, we believe that the researchers who tested Yb are not justified to accuse Chu of misconduct. After all, Chu could have accused them of misconduct, since they had tried to take advantage of a breach in the confidentiality of the reviewing process. Could it be

Chu's genius attempt to pre-emptively overthrow accusations for scientific fraud? Could it be an effort to mock those that were about to steal his results? We cannot know and from this point on the whole discussion becomes highly speculative. The fact that the Yb-based materials revealed high T_C superconductivity is, most possibly, a completely coincidental event.

Should *PRL*'s reviewers be held responsible for a breach of confidentiality? We believe that the reviewers should be the last ones to be held responsible, since Chu had a word on their selection, so they should have been reliable researchers. In addition, it is certain that both reviewers should have felt quite exposed in the eyes of the chief editor and, in this respect, they would have refrained from revealing any kind of confidential information. Should groups studying Yb-based materials or PRL itself be made responsible for misconduct? We do not know the way the Yb-based "ghost" material found its way to the rival groups. It could have been from another person at *PRL*, perhaps someone with secretarial duties, or it could be just a rumour unintentionally escaped from a reviewer or from Chu's alleged "informer". Finally, we should also consider that the study of Yb-based materials could have been just another coincidence.

7.5.4   Connection to the PRO-RES Toolbox

This section is mostly related to the PRO-RES toolbox via the question: *"What were the OUTCOMES of the research?"*, focusing on how were the research/analysis findings reported, shared and/or disseminated. The issues concerning the dissemination paths Chu followed or did not follow have been commented in the previous section. The toolbox sets some additional queries that go beyond the above discussion. Specifically, it requires a response to questions like whether any form of 'impact assessment' was performed, and whether any kind of evaluation of the outcomes was conducted or was planned to take place. Both issues are related to the organisation of research beyond the conduct of the original experiments.

Chu pushed the frontiers of superconductors with the limited resources he had at his disposal, because several potential applications of high T_C superconductors were already known. However, besides this horizon scanning exercise that was triggering research in superconductors for decades, a specific breakthrough was needed to be based on a sound impact assessment analysis. As for the evaluation of the outcomes, this was done meticulously but necessarily at the low technology readiness level of the ongoing research that was of fundamental character and strictly within the walls of Chu's laboratory.

Industrial laboratories, as we will see in the last section of this chapter, had succeeded in producing real demonstrators for the computer industry, meaning that they were working at a technology readiness level of four or five, significantly higher than that of Chu. We can assume that these laboratories, backed by private companies, would have already been in the process of making an impact assessment, since they had a very specific commercial product to produce. Chu, working in isolation in the context of an academic research laboratory, could not have made progress beyond the level of fundamental research, at least within the extremely tight duration of the race for the superconductor.

7.6 The Darker Gatekeepers

Such an important scientific advance, with a potential enormous technological impact, could not have been left unnoticed by people outside the scientific community. According to Hazen (1990), Chu was summoned to Washington, D.C. by a panel of high-ranking officials, responsible for the Strategic Defense Initiative (SDI),[2] commonly known as "Star Wars". Chu had already elaborated a number of potential military applications of his discovery. For example, the new high T_C superconductor could store huge amounts of energy, could be used to produce hypersensitive sensors for infra-red radiation or render lightweight computers a reality. High T_C superconductors could be a key discovery for the SDI, in which Chu saw an opportunity for vast amounts of funding. Chu presented himself in front of four people on 13 February 1987 (i.e. BEFORE his famous paper was published).

The meeting very quickly took a grim character. These four people asked Chu to give them all the results of his publicly funded research. Chu refused to give any details, despite the fact that he was actually warned that he may have to give explanations about his refusal to people with enormous power, like the president of the National Science Foundation and people that were consulting the government on scientific issues. When the people in Washington were convinced that Chu would not reveal details of his discovery, they brought the meeting to an abrupt end.

One thing was clear to Chu: he was neither going to ask nor receive financial support from the SDI programme.

7.6.1 List of Questions

- Are there grounds on which one could agree with the demands of the SDI people?
- Do you think that a scientist should take a critical stand when she/he recognizes a *Dual Use* potential for her/his research?

7.6.2 Terms from the PRO-RES Glossary

Academic Freedom, Conflict of interest, Dual use, Independence of Research.

---

[2] A program initiated on 23 March 1983, under US President Ronald Reagan. The aim was to develop a sophisticated anti-ballistic missile system, in order to prevent missile attacks from other countries, specifically the Soviet Union.

7.6.3   Comments

Chu was conducting research that was not funded by the military. He was struggling to secure funding for his small research group, since he was working in a field that did not promise any kind of breakthrough until late 1986. When Chu was summoned to Washington, he met people working for the military establishment. Their basic demand was for the complete results of his research for those to be used for purely military purposes. If we leave aside the persistence of the demands and the non-cordial way Chu was treated in Washington, according to Hazen (1990), a basic question is if those people had the right to make any kind of demands on an independent researcher.

It goes without saying that a unilateral decision from SDI's side to seize Chu's invention would be a flagrant breach of academic freedom and the independence of research. Chu seemingly, had he accepted, would have continued to work on a classified project, considering the nature of the SDI. As a result, the potentially enormous societal impact of high T_C superconductors in civil applications would have been lost, at least for a considerable amount of time. As a result, we believe that Chu made the right decision not to hand off his research into the hands of the military establishment.

However, the reasons behind the rejection of the "offer" from the SDI people has to be discussed a little further. Chu was not against military applications of his research, since he had already made a list of such, presumably as a means to secure funding. We do not know if Chu had discussed the issue with the University of Houston administration before he appeared in Washington or if any cooperation with SDI could create a conflict of interest with the patent submission his University had already made. Chu's rejection might have more to do with his worries that he would lose academic credit and control over the future planning of his high T_C superconductivity research.

Perhaps he had seen the whole SDI challenge from the perspective of a scientist from China working in the USA. That could mean that as soon as he had communicated all sensitive information to SDI, he would have been probably transformed into a "straw man", having access only to low security level research, if at all, while the real research would carry on at the high security echelons of SDI by American researchers. If it is assumed that the rejection of the SDI offer was incentivized not by pacifism but by a desire to maximize personal professional benefit does it have the same "ethical quality"? Pacifist or not Chu did not hand over his research to SDI; but does he merit praise for that?

Another question could be, even if he had rejected for reasons of pacifism, would that be a response that should be viewed positively? This raises a very thorny issue: that of the responsibility of a researcher who works on a project with Dual Use potential. Doing research on a project where results can have civil and military applications means that the risk of misuse or abuse of research results is considerable, i.e. there is a possibility of malevolent use of research. Should a researcher working in a University deny involvement in Dual Use research altogether or strive to put all necessary safeguards in place so that her/his research will not be used by terrorist groups or rogue governments? Before the reader responds we should mention that most researchers do not have the appropriate expertise to realize the Dual Use nature or potential of the research they are involved in.

7.6.4   Connection to the PRO-RES Toolbox

Again, this section is mostly related to the PRO-RES toolbox via "*What were the OUTCOMES of the research?*" The issues concerning the dissemination paths Chu followed or did not follow have been commented on extensively. What has not yet been commented on, but is brought forward by the Toolbox, is whether Chu derived or gave any kind of policy advice. Actually, Chu experienced the reverse effect: policy makers actually asked him to inform them about the progress of his, seemingly, ground-breaking research, and to convince him to give them the control of his research for exclusively military purposes. We do not know what offer was made to him, but we do know that Chu was clearly taken aback by the insistence of the SDI people. This is a case where a technological breakthrough finds an immediate area of application; this is mainly because Chu's achievement was a long and highly anticipated scientific progress.

7.7   The Aftermath

All the major scientists who took part in the discovery of high T_C superconductors participated in the so-called "*Woodstock of Physics*"; this refers to the marathon session of the American Physical Society's meeting on 18 March 1987, which featured 51 presentations about the science of high T_C superconductors. Bednorz and Müller were there, as well as Chu, Kitazawa, Zhao and several other scientists who played a crucial or not so crucial role in the discovery and interpretation of the phenomenon of superconductivity in oxide systems. There were also scientists from industrial laboratories who had already succeeded not only in producing a high T_C superconductor, but also in producing actual demonstrators for the computer industry. There, in front of an enthusiastic audience, all recent and current advances, covered until then under a cloud of secrecy, were openly presented to the scientific community and to the public, since the event was covered by mass media.

Chu was acknowledged as one of the main players of the progress that had just taken place. However, the path to glory did not reach the heights he had perhaps dreamt of. The Nobel Prize in Physics for 1987 was awarded jointly to Bednorz and Müller "*for their important break-through in the discovery of superconductivity in ceramic materials*", as it was described in the press release of the Swedish Academy of Sciences. For some critics, this decision was based on the wish of the Swedish Academy of Sciences not to be involved in the competition over who was the first to discover high T_C superconductivity and, perhaps, a delicate way to avoid the complications with publication ethics where Chu had been involved, intentionally or unintentionally.

7.7.1   List of Questions

- Should the Swedish Academy take into account issues of research ethics, apart from the strictly technical ones, when deciding on the Nobel Prize laureates?

7.7.2   Terms from the PRO-RES Glossary

Questionable Research Practices, Research misconduct.

7.7.3   Comments

We do not know if the Swedish Academy nominated Bednorz and Müller in an effort to circumvent the debate over the *PRL* issue. It should be mentioned, though that if the scientific community believed that Chu committed research misconduct or applied Questionable Research Practices, then the institutional or National Research Ethics Committee should have conducted a formal investigation. No such action was taken, at least based on the information presented by Hazen (1990). This could lead to the conclusion that either Chu's deeds were deemed honest, or the scientific community wanted the issue to just fade away. However, this will probably remain unresolved not because it is a case of unprecedented difficulty but because it created an atmosphere of embarrassment.

7.8   Epilogue

One of the fundamental statements of the PRO-RES Accord is that, "*As individuals and institutions involved in commissioning, funding, sponsoring or conducting research, collecting or using evidence for policymaking, we aim to be as transparent as possible on how the high quality of that evidence is assured and will flag up any potential conflicts of interest.*" As described, this case study, chronicled by Hazen in "*The Breakthrough: The Race for the Superconductor*" (1990), brings forth a whole array of departures from the above statement. Chu conducted research under a thick cloud of secrecy that he was reluctant to compromise even when the time for the assessment of his findings came, i.e. during the review process for his ground-breaking publication. This is the "crux" of the whole case, in the sense that it embodies specific ethical dilemmas within the research enterprise. Chu and *PRL*'s chief editor were entangled in a delicate balance between following the standards of publication ethics and being pragmatic about the possibility of leaks in the review and editorial process.

Perhaps Chu could have defined his actions as being "as transparent as possible" in the unusual situation in which he found himself, where policy makers had already set a plan to exploit Chu's research before they contacted him. It is improbable that Chu could have envisioned the needs of SDI, which was a highly classified project, while we do not know if the SDI people were aware of the progress Chu had made up until February 1987 or if they had any kind of knowledge of the reliability of Chu's research. In addition, the SDI people were seemingly absolutely unconcerned about the manifold conflicts of interest that might have curbed Chu's intention for collaboration.

The "race for the superconductor", due to its uniqueness that stems from its complexity and from the extreme character of the ethical dilemmas it evoked, is an excellent, albeit forgotten, case study from the area of Natural Sciences. We were greatly aided in our analysis by the resources of the PRO-RES toolbox and the statements that make up the "Accord". We believe that PRO-RES brings a valuable array of tools with which ethical dilemmas can be acknowledged and provides a structured collection of high-level recommendations that urge the researcher and policy maker to ask the right questions in order to create an environment that facilitates evidence-based decisions.

References

Ashcroft, Neil and David Mermin. 1976. *Solid state physics*. Saunders College Publishing.

Baker, Monya. 2016. 1,500 scientists lift the lid on reproducibility. *Nature* 533: 452–454.

Baker, Monya, and Elie Dolgin. 2017. Cancer reproducibility project releases first results. *Nature* 541: 269–270.

Bednorz, Georg, and Alex Müller. 1986. Possible high T_C superconductivity in the Ba-La-Cu-O system. *Zeitschrift Für Physik B Condensed Matter* 64: 189–193.

Bohannon, John. 2015. Many psychology papers fail replication tests. *Science* 349: 910–911.

Chu, C.W., P.H. Hor, R.L. Meng, L. Gao, and Z.J. Huang. 1987a. Superconductivity at 52.5 K in the lanthanum-barium-copper-oxide system. *Science* 235: 567–569.

Chu, C.W., P.H. Hor, R.L. Meng, L. Gao, Z.J. Huang, and Y.Q. Wang. 1987b. Evidence for *super-conductivity above 40 K* in the La-Ba-Cu-O compound system. *Physical Review Letters* 58: 405–407.

Hazen, R.M. 1988. *The breakthrough: The race for the superconductor*. Summit Books/Simon & Schuster.

Hazen R.M. 1990. Η ΡΗΞΗ - Η κούρσα της υπεραγωγιμότητας. ΤΡΟΧΑΛΙΑ editions ISBN: 960-7022-11-4.

Ioannidis, J.P.A. 2005. Why most published research findings are false. *PLOS Medicine* 2: e124. https://doi.org/10.1371/journal.pmed.0020124.

Iqbal, Shareen A., Joshua D. Wallach, Muin J. Khoury, Sheri D. Schoully, and John P. A. Ioannidis. 2016. Reproducible research practices and transparency across the biomedical literature. *PLoS Biology* 14: e1002333. https://doi.org/10.1371/journal.pbio.1002333.

van Delft, Dirk. 2007. *Freezing physics: Heike Kamerlingh Onnes and the quest for cold*. Royal Netherlands Academy of Arts and Sciences.

Wu, M.K., J.R. Ashburn, C.J. Torng, P.H. Hor, R.L. Meng, L. Gao, Z.J. Huang, Y.Q. Wang, and C.W. Chu. 1987. Superconductivity at 93 K in a new mixed-phase Y-Ba-Cu-O compound system at ambient pressure. *Physical Review Letters* 58: 908–910.

Chapter 8
The UK Wave Power Project: Salter's Duck

Ron Iphofen

Abstract This chapter outlines what happened to research into a new and unorthodox energy technology that could have helped displace traditional energy supply methods by extracting energy from the waves at sea. The project received funding filtered via the administrative structure of the traditional and competing energy system—nuclear power. The funding source constantly delayed and obstructed the supply of funds making day-to-day operations difficult to manage and the results of the research were assessed by experts who worked within the old technology and so had vested and conflicting interests. This case offers an example of trying to do research with integrity while the researchers were placed in a 'no win' situation. Considerable ethical reflection is required to fully understand the context in which the research had to be conducted. The lessons are apt for innovative disruptive technologies that are framed by political, economic and ideological constraints. Those constraints, together with the evident research misconduct that took place, can only be described as sabotage. Again, such actions must be understood in terms of the balance of many interests, most of which failed to live up to standards of professional research integrity.

Keywords Wave power · Stephen Salter · Renewable energy research · Transparency · Funding agencies

8.1 Introduction: The Case in Outline

In the early 1970s in the United Kingdom (UK) and elsewhere research into 'alternative' energy sources was growing partly as a consequence of emergent theories of global warming and the oil crisis. The latter arose out of the Arab producers of the Organization of Petroleum Exporting Countries (OPEC) putting in place an embargo on oil exports to the United States in October 1973 and threatening to cut back overall production 25% (Udall 1973). Any research into a new, untested and

R. Iphofen (✉)
Independent Research Consultant, La Rochelle, France
e-mail: ron.iphofen@gmail.com

© The Author(s) 2022
D. O'Mathúna and R. Iphofen (eds.), *Ethics, Integrity and Policymaking*, Research Ethics Forum 9, https://doi.org/10.1007/978-3-031-15746-2_8

unorthodox energy technology that could displace traditional and polluting energy supply methods required at least some realistic start-up funding. Given the size of funding needed the most likely source for such untested technologies would be governmental. The new technology discussed in this case study was one method for extracting energy from sea waves: the Edinburgh Wave Power Project led by Professor Stephen Salter who was head of the Department of Mechanical Engineering at Edinburgh University (ERA 2021).

Given that our concerns for this book relate to the ethical issues that can arise in such situations a series of questions immediately present themselves: What are the immediate consequences of giving funding to new technologies that could undermine previous (traditional) ways of producing energy? What range of 'interests' are involved? What broader policies influence the research and the views of funders and government? Does it matter who funds the research? Is there too much opportunity for misconduct depending on how funds are disbursed? And does it matter who analyses the results? These are the kind of questions addressed in the following case study.

At this point I must declare an interest of my own. I am a supporter of alternative energy technologies that could reduce all forms of environmental pollution and, thereby, help minimize human-induced global warming. More specifically the origins of such a view lie in my experience with the Wave Power Project itself from 1974 to 1977. My wife was then a Personal Assistant (P.A.) to Stephen Salter and told me of her frustration in getting the main source of funding to deliver the correct funding in good time. She constantly had to phone the funder and was regularly offered unreasonable excuses for delays—the consequence of which were that the salaries for the young engineering researchers were rarely paid in time and money for materials always delayed. Such a tactic seemed problematic to me at the time until she explained the funding was disbursed by the UK Atomic Energy Authority— one of the 'old' polluting technologies that alternative energy projects were directly challenging. Perhaps this was a rationale for the tactic that could only be described as 'undermining'?

For my college teaching post at the time I was tasked with delivering a series of lectures of a 'general' nature and thought something on alternative energy technologies would be of interest to my experienced mature students—who were all 'older adults' entering further and higher education for the first time. I invited both the Wave Power Project and the Atomic Energy Authority to come and give a talk about the merits of their approach. The Wave Power Project sent one of their researchers who gave an informed and stimulating talk about the balance in terms of cost and effectiveness of different energy sources and showed some photographs to illustrate their ongoing work. The Atomic Energy Authority sent no-one but delivered (at their considerable expense) boxes of hundreds of reprinted articles to be distributed freely for the benefit of my students. All the articles were in support of nuclear energy without providing a balanced perspective on the controversies surrounding nuclear energy. I cannot say I suffered a 'confirmation bias' prior to those experiences, but it certainly grew subsequently as my suspicions of at least some lack of fairness in funding were aroused.

These details, in relation to a specific research activity, illustrates that 'who funds and how?' raises a series of ethical questions along with whether a balanced assessment of alternative options—in any field of research—is vital to honest, reliable and trustworthy research. Trust in the funding source becomes part of transparency of practice that can help the public and policymakers decide on the best ways of proceeding with an innovative, and potentially challenging, technology.

8.2 More Background and Context

Research into marine wave power really began with Salter's experiments using a dynamically shaped float (the 'Duck') that linked via a spine to a series of other floating 'Ducks' which bobbed up and down in the waves. The Duck was a 300-tonne floating canister designed to drive a generator from the motion of bobbing up and down on waves like a duck. It is still regarded as the most efficient of any wave power system produced, converting up to 80% of the wave energy to electricity which was to be then cabled ashore. All the experiments were successful until 1982 when the work suddenly stopped. Salter (2016) provides a full discussion of both the key technical issues and the emergent governance problems.

The funding problem arose from the control of all renewable energy research—not just wave power—during the 1970s and 1980s coming from an organisation that was part of the United Kingdom Atomic Energy Authority. The Department of Energy's research and development advisory council (ACORD) operated at long range from all the projects and its staff was recruited largely from the nuclear and the depletable energy industries. In other words, wave power research was funded and controlled by the regulators of the nuclear, coal and gas industries.

By 1982, an independent consultant reported that the Duck could be expected, with further development, to produce electricity at a cost of around 5.5 pence per kW-h, which would have been a price competitive with nuclear power. Clive Grove-Palmer, a respected Department engineer seconded to work on the Duck project, estimated that the cost could be decreased to around 3 pence per kW-h. ACORD met in 1982, excluded Grove-Palmer and his findings, and instead accepted a secret report, prepared by a unit based at British Atomic Energy Authority headquarters, claiming that wind power had more immediate commercial possibilities than wave power, and research funds should be shifted to it. At the same time the Department of Energy, which was packed with nuclear supporters, had instructed ACORD to reduce its renewable energy research budget from £14 million to £11 million. The Department was then spending around £200 million on nuclear research (all data from GLW 1992).

The wave power researchers were not given sight of the report on which ACORD based its decision to denigrate and stop their work until eight months later. Then, in January 1983, a research unit based at the Atomic Energy Authority came out with another report concealing the highly favourable figures for the Duck by averaging them in with figures for all other wave power projects. This gave a non-commercial figure of 8–12 pence per kW-h. "Opponents of the project then produced figures overestimating capital costs by a factor of ten, massively underestimating the reliability of undersea cables, and claiming that in mass production each Duck would cost about the same as one prototype" (GLW 1992).

To illustrate the nature of the sabotage employed, the following is from the written evidence to the House of Lords Select Committee by A. Gordon Senior an independent consultant appointed by Rendell Palmer and Tritton (RPT) responsible for reporting specifically on the Duck project to the Department of Energy: "My final draft of these sections was submitted in May 1983. I expected a response from RPT within days to discuss these consistent with our established practice. When this was not forthcoming I telephoned the RPT Project Manager to be told that the report had been completed, was to be submitted that night and could not be discussed. When pressed I was told that the conclusions had been altered. When I asked for a copy to examine what changes had been made I was told that no copy had been allocated to me and that copies were in short supply. When I pressed harder I was offered a copy on loan. I found that most of the text of the report was as I had drafted but the key conclusions had indeed been changed and even reversed. I objected and asked for my views to be made known to the DEn (Dept. of Energy) but was told that this could not be done and that I was bound by client confidentiality to RPT not to reveal my disagreement. I was also advised not to have further contact with the device team" (HL Paper 88, 204). The extent of the dissembling, dishonesty and fraudulence beggars belief.

The seconded engineer Grove-Palmer took early retirement as a result of the decision. "I resigned … because they asked me to write the obituary of wave power. There was no way I could do that … We were just ready to do the final year of development and then go to sea" (GLW 1992).

After a long campaign to save the project, Professor Salter's team was forced to disperse in early 1987. "We must not waste another 15 years and dissipate the high motivation of another generation of young engineers", wrote Salter in a memorandum to the House of Lords committee on renewable energy. "We must stop using grossly different assessment methods in a rat race between technologies at widely differing stages of their development. We must find a way of reporting accurate results to decision makers and have decision makers with enough technical knowledge to spot data massage if it occurs. I believe that this will be possible only if the control of renewable energy projects is completely removed from nuclear influences."[1] This is a plea for transparency, fairness and accurate comparative analyses of the competing sources.

This brief account makes it very clear just how conflicting the vested interests were. Having experts drawn from a competing energy source to cast judgement on innovative research that could challenge their own professional interests is a recipe for disaster and lacks fairness. The disparity in research funding in itself undermines any equality in allowing a realistic challenge from wave power. The lack of independent peer review and honest comparative analysis of the cost effectiveness of different

---

[1] This and all Salter's quotes are taken from HL Paper 88.

energy sources immediately arouses suspicion of underhand behaviour. The decision to pervert the figures supplied by the independent consultant would today be regarded as fraudulent and a challenge to modern standards of research integrity. Selfish vested interest may not be enough to account for how these actions could have been allowed. Lack of transparency at the time would make it difficult to mount any public challenge of such research misbehaviour. But we also need to consider if there could be any valid reasons to promote nuclear power at the expense of green alternatives.

8.3 The Researchers' Views

Professor Salter gave the following assessment of reasons for the failure of the Project to a House of Commons Parliamentary Select Committee in 2001: "If I had to supply reasons for the failure of the first UK wave programme I would cite over-optimism, the attempt to make very big (2GW) power stations and to assess infant devices too quickly. The programme was properly supported and enthusiastically led from 1976 to 1983, a period of only seven years, and then entered a very unhappy phase where researchers felt that they were always on the defensive. An account of this has been given to a Committee of another place (HL Paper 88 1988, 21 June 1988 page 178 and 190–206) and it does not, at present, seem helpful to repeat it here" (STC 2001).

The Select Committee asked what role wave and tidal stream energy should have in the Government's renewable energy strategy? Should they have a higher priority?

Salter's answer subtly shows recognition of the disguised vested interests that caused his early work to be sabotaged: "This must depend on whether the Government and its civil servants really want renewable energy to succeed or whether they want to appear to be supporting a programme but really want it to fail. Over the years many of the officials with whom we dealt certainly seemed to want success but this often proved to be a dangerous career move. I must warn the Committee that this danger is not confined to officials. There was a Commons Energy Committee which looked into renewables in 1992. A copy of my evidence (pages 62–68 of volume III) is attached. One of the Committee's recommendations was the resurrection of the wave energy programme. The Energy Committee was immediately disbanded!"

This clearly suggests that a hidden underlying policy was governing decisions about allowing successful green energy competition more than ten years later and one would have to wonder if that applies even today—but how would we know?

Salter continued to the Committee: "Always there seems to be a layer, or indeed layers, of senior people with negative views about renewables and the power to make them stick. This power seems to be inversely related to technical knowledge of the subject or technology in general. If the concerns about carbon levels, global warming and long-term supplies of fossil fuels are well founded, then the Government policy should be that every possible renewable source should be thoroughly researched to the point that it could rapidly be employed at some stage in the future. The demonstration of this capability would do much to limit the dangers of a manipulated market for oil or gas and could be regarded as part of a nation's defences." This observation becomes particularly apt in the current climate, with the Russian invasion of Ukraine and the consequent disruption of energy supplies as a result of the sanctions imposed on Russia by a number of governments. So, as Salter observed, "The costs of a vigorous research programme are very small compared with the total spending on fuel or the possible future consequences of having insufficient energy supplies. The spin-off in unexpected directions has, so far, been quite sufficient to justify what has been spent. Diversity between renewable sources with different availability reduces the problems caused by lack of firmness of supply. This could be further reduced by the use of renewable sources for the manufacture of hydrogen, methanol, ammonia or even potable water" (HL Paper 88, 1988).

In an era when Government constantly reassures us that they are 'following the science' we have to wonder if that operates in only some spheres of influence and how much in other spheres is kept hidden. Then and now officials (elected and/or appointed) are clearly in a position to override scientific findings and can get away with it due to the impossibility of gaining full transparency for public awareness of why certain policy decisions are taken. There appears to have been (and still is?) a group of people at senior levels with the power to impose their own agenda—a lack of transparency permits a high degree of dishonesty. There is a question of whether policy responsibilities should be kept separate from those of the scientists/researchers. They are not after all elected to their position of responsibility and their responsibilities are to science and not to the electorate. On the other hand, that would suggest that scientists have no responsibility to society and such a view hardly holds water today in light of all the work done in the name of RRI (Responsible Research and Innovation). The question then must be how can scientists fairly represent the benefits of their work to those who must take the policy decisions? Evidently a fair, honest and transparent assessment of the relative merits of, in this case, alternative energy supplies that leads to a clear appraisal of the available options and their consequences would have been the most effective way of proceeding and in the best interests of society. We must still ask if there is any way in which both the scant unequal funding and the deliberate sabotage of findings could be ethically justified.

8.4   Lessons Learned: How Should National Funding for New Technologies Be Managed?

Professor Salter's further responses to House of Lords Committee's questions (STC 2001) offer lessons:

> ...Private investors must protect their investment by secrecy in a way that is totally foreign to academics, even if a large fraction of the money is coming from public sources. There are even stronger motives for secrecy following poor productivity or the loss of a prototype. Mistakes will then be repeated by others. It does not have to be like this. Following an aircraft accident there is a very expensive investigation with the most detailed information supplied

to and carefully studied by the entire industry. This should be an obligation in return for receipt of public money.

If such an approach can be adopted in the aviation industry, where one might argue the risks of harm are likely to be higher and the investment costs fairly similar then why not in energy supplies? Strict central/ministerial direction would violate the independence of research funding councils. "…This independence is important because there is also documentary evidence that an official from the Energy Technology Support Unit (ETSU) at Harwell (then part of the United Kingdom Atomic Energy Authority) tried hard… to discourage support for wave energy from Brussels. Over-strict co-ordination stifles original ideas. I am, therefore, on balance in favour of open published consultation between independent bodies and a degree of anarchy."

Once again transparency was avoided, attempts to influence European policy one-sided, and Salter's 'anarchy' seems to amount to a plea for fair competition to avoid the dirigiste errors of either monopoly capitalism or state control. However, Salter illustrates the dilemmas with a specific example: he sees "…a serious co-ordination problem concerning test tank facilities[2] which I would like to draw to the attention of your Committee. It concerns test facilities for wave energy research, which I regard as essential and which are expensive enough to have to be nationally coordinated. …Funding for most academic work, now including waves, is the responsibility of the Engineering and Physical Sciences Research Council, which is given money by Government but notionally makes independent decisions. I have some evidence that this independence was not complete when, in 1986, a proposal for work on wave energy was rejected on the grounds that it was not strategic, as defined by the Renewable Energy Advisory Group set up by the DTI" (Department for Trade and Industry).

One could hardly challenge the rights, indeed responsibility, of governments to direct 'strategic' research and funding. But once again should that be decided entirely 'behind the scenes'? Perhaps the public and the researchers should not be kept in the dark about such decisions and, in the case of the latter, undermine their work and careers by permitting them to work in fields that were not to be supported for hidden 'strategic' reasons. The strategic issue here surely relates to the mutual dependence of nuclear power and nuclear weaponry suggesting that full transparency about such sensitive matters might be unrealistic. Ultimately one suspects that the then Government could not allow nuclear power to 'fail' relative to alternative sources in order to maintain adequate fuel supplies for nuclear weaponry. But given that the maintenance of nuclear arms was an open governmental policy, why not be open about the inequality of treatment for the different energy sources? An obvious answer might be that the public, and interested pressure groups in particular, might find their nuclear disarmament perspective strengthened by the knowledge that the nuclear arms race was a factor in blocking the development of renewable energy sources that could deliver cheaper electricity that was less polluting and less likely to contribute

---

[2] Test tanks are the scale models within which alternative wave energy-capturing devices could be compared.

to global warming. Defending continuing nuclear arms was a difficult enough policy without shooting themselves in the foot with admitting to blocking better energy sources.

Although this particular case happened some time ago it is interesting to note that the determination to hide the true costs of nuclear power has been sustained even after the turn of the century—for example, in the UK in 2003 a Green Party local government councillor was dismissed for a period from council duties for breaching confidentiality. The breach was over a discussion that was to be 'kept secret' over a deferment of payment of business rates that would cost the council £18,000, and the same had occurred in six other local authorities. No other commercial businesses would have been accorded this privilege. The British Government had recently removed the public interest clause from the councillors' code of duties which would have protected the councillor's duty to disclose (Dowding 2003).

So many ethical issues arise in trying to find the balance for new technology research between 'national coordination' and what Salter called 'anarchy'. Given the strategic issues raised above the question then becomes how an effective balance can be struck between central government funding, private investment and 'independent' research councils—each with their specific vested and possibly conflicting interests. Of course this does not only apply to energy research but research into any new, disruptive technologies that challenge governmental strategic decisions— it just becomes more complicated when those strategies remain undisclosed. One might argue that, in the interests of democracy, government should retain the ultimate control—of both private enterprise and research funding councils. The questions then are—how much control, should it be limited and, if so, how?

Clearly the answers to those questions must be contextual. It will depend upon just what the topics of interest are and precisely the kind of 'disruption' the innovative technologies are likely to create. Energy research is clearly such an area—even excluding the nuclear arms issue. The threats to coal, gas and oil, regardless of their inevitably limited supply, in the short term, threatens to undermine a major material and socioeconomic infrastructure. However, in the long term, it is obvious these energy sources will be depleted in a short enough timespan to require a centrally coordinated, probably international, plan to replace them with alternative, renewable and non-polluting sources. Evidence can be found for such an approach within the European Union.[3] It is also important to note that my argument in this case is not about whether or not nuclear power should be ditched in favour of alternative, 'greener', technologies. Even ecologists argue for a sustainable nuclear industry on the grounds that the alternatives are incapable of meeting growing power demands (Jancovici 2021). Rather it is about how that debate should be conducted and how the evidence is produced and used.

Our remaining concern is how we can be assured that any future policies draw on ethical evidence in making such crucial decisions. The evidence from the Wave

[3] Directive 2009/28/EC of the European Parliament and of the Council of 23 April 2009 on the promotion of the use of energy from renewable sources and amending and subsequently repealing Directives 2001/77/EC and 2003/30/EC.

Power Project case study suggests that peer review processes should be independent, entirely separated from funding and strategic issues. That evidence should be delivered transparently to the key decision takers along with any available appraisal of options, and the decisions taken should be open, especially if they are governed by strategic factors. The public and scientists have a right to know what the strategies are of those who they elected.

8.5 Summary Lessons Learned: Guidance for Policymakers

Professor Michael Davis of the Illinois Institute of Technology, Chicago, has made some interesting observations about ethics in engineering research which illustrate some of the problems that faced the Duck Project: "Engineering research takes place in at least four domains: the laboratory, the pilot, digital models, and 'the field.' In the laboratory, engineering research most resembles research in physics, chemistry, or biology. Issues concerning accuracy, truthfulness, crediting, and the like are much the same in engineering as in the sciences. The chief distinctive ethical issue in engineering research in the lab is that the research should seek to improve the material condition of humanity, not just seek knowledge for its own sake. There is no 'pure engineering.' … In the field, the ethical issues in engineering research most resemble those in public health. For example, engineers should keep good records of complaints about their products; have procedures for quickly identifying threats to the public health, safety, or welfare; and have procedures in place for responding appropriately. Research in engineering is continuous with the practice of engineering" (Davis 2020, 967–968).

Policymakers and regulators have a responsibility to consider how best to manage emergent technologies in light of strategic contradictions. What may be seen as 'anarchy' from one perspective, may be legitimately viewed as 'healthy competition' from another. For example, in the later 1990s there was a distinct drive towards the globally coordinated regulation of genetics research—the 'risks' estimated to be so high that such uniform standards were seen as a necessary alternative to a dangerous anarchy (see HGP 2021). Little consideration was given to the possibility of allowing diverse national regulation leading to a 'regulatory competition' which could then be studied to assess what sort of regime worked best rather than having global standards imposed by individual unaccountable bioethicists.

Thus Salter's Duck illustrates the problem of balancing independence in research, free markets in technological developments and governmental dirigisme. The project received funding via the administrative structure of the traditional and 'competing' technical system. Funding was constantly delayed and then results of the research assessed by 'experts' who worked within the old technology—and, crucially, they knowingly distorted the findings. Centralised coordination can stultify genuine innovation if researchers are prevented from pursuing their own promising lines of thought. The possibility of 'dead ends' and the 'waste' of scarce funding resources might have to be risked for exciting and productive innovation to win through.

The major ethical lesson arising out of these observations is that though transparency in governmental actions may seem the most moral course, that may be balanced against strategic requirements that ensure societal safety and stability. How to identify such a rationale against 'political expediency' remains moot.

References

Davis, M. 2020. Engineering research and ethics. In *Handbook of research ethics and scientific integrity*, ed. Ron Iphofen, 968–981. Switzerland: Springer Nature.

Dowding, G. 2003. Going public. *The Guardian*, 19 November 2013.

ERA. 2021. The Edinburgh Wave Power Project. *Edinburgh Research Archive*. https://era.ed.ac.uk/handle/1842/23407. Accessed 31 Dec 2021.

GLW. 1992. The untimely death of Salter's Duck, *Green Left Weekly*, Issue 64. July 29. https://www.greenleft.org.au/content/untimely-death-salters-duck. Accessed 31 Aug 2021.

HGP (The Human Genome Project). 2021. National Human Genome Research Institute. https://www.genome.gov/human-genome-project/What. Accessed 31 Aug 2021.

HL Paper 88. 1988. *House of lords, Select Committee on the European Communities, alternative energy sources (report with evidence)*. London: Her Majesty's Stationery Office.

Jancovici, J.-M. 2021. I am an ecologist and believe in the power of nuclear. *The Connexion*, May 15.

Physics and Ethics Education Project. Salter's Duck. http://www.peep.ac.uk/content/1113.0.html. Accessed 31 Dec 2021.

Salter, S. 2016. Wave energy: Nostalgic Ramblings, future hopes and heretical suggestions. *Journal of Ocean Engineering and Marine Energy* 2: 399–428. https://doi.org/10.1007/s40722-016-0057-3.

STC (Science and Technology Committee of the House of Commons). 2001. Minutes of evidence, taken before the science and technology committee, March 14. https://publications.parliament.uk/pa/cm200001/cmselect/cmsctech/291/1031401.htm. Accessed 31 Aug 2021.

Udall, M.K. 1973. How congress planned to solve the 1970s energy crisis. *The New Republic*, June 16. https://newrepublic.com/article/118918/how-congress-planned-solve-1970s-energy-crisis. Accessed 31 Aug 2021.

Chapter 9
Ethics in Space: The Case for Future Space Exploration

Emmanuel Detsis

Abstract The coming decades will see humans setting foot on the Moon once more and possibly Mars. However, current radiation exposure standards for long duration spaceflight do not allow for such missions. This chapter gives an overview of the discussion in the US and NASA, regarding the way forward and outlines important recommendations that were presented to NASA from the National Academies of Science, Engineering and Medicine in 2021. The ethical issues regarding human spaceflight and radiation exposure are highlighted and examined.

Keywords Ethics of human space flight · Space exploration

9.1 Introduction

The images of the Apollo landing on the Moon are one of the most iconic of the twentieth century. Neil Armstrong's "one small step for man, one giant leap for mankind" inspired millions of people around the world, helped boost the U.S geopolitical image around the globe and was the winning aspect of the US-Soviet "Space Race". Understandably, the Apollo program (11 total missions, 6 Moon landings and 12 astronauts walking on the Moon) was and still is the crowning achievement of human space flight. However, the program ended in 1972, and since then, humans in space have remained very close to Earth indeed. Operating in Low Earth Orbit (LEO), mostly within space stations such as Skylab (US), Mir (Soviet Union and then Russia), the International Space Station (US/Russia/EU/Japan/Canada) and the Tiangong-1, 2 and 3 (China). These stations circle the Earth at orbits between 350 and 450 km.

However, we are entering once again an era of space exploration beyond Earth, with the Moon as a steppingstone and Mars as the ultimate destination. Plans for these kinds of missions have always existed but it seems that the 2020–2030 decade will once again see humans on the Moon, or soon within the decades after. These

E. Detsis (✉)
European Science Foundation, Strasbourg, France
e-mail: edetsis@esf.org

© The Author(s) 2022
D. O'Mathúna and R. Iphofen (eds.), *Ethics, Integrity and Policymaking*, Research Ethics Forum 9, https://doi.org/10.1007/978-3-031-15746-2_9

plans for the Moon have gone now beyond the planning phase and are now being "operationalized", with NASA having signed the "Artemis Accords"[1] and other space agencies adapting their own space programs or parts thereof for operations in the lunar vicinity and/or surface, in partnership with NASA or concurrently, as is the Chinese/Russian plan for an International Lunar Research Station on the Moon, as announced at the Global Space Exploration conference on June 16, 2021.

Obviously, there is a plethora of questions to be answered regarding the "how?", encompassing the myriad of technical issues to be solved and worked out in order to make a Moon or Mars landing feasible. There are also several questions regarding "why?", that have to do with the purpose of landing humans on an extra-terrestrial surface, being either scientific or political in nature.

However, this case study will not delve into these aspects, but rather focus on the issue of whether sending humans to another celestial body is an ethical thing to do, and how space agencies currently deal with the ethical issue that the mere presence of humans in space puts them in harm's way.

9.2   Space Exploration and Effects on Humans

"Space is hard" is a common saying amongst people working in the space industry. It signifies the complicated issues surrounding space travel, an issue that is also reflected on the cost of space missions. Space travel beyond LEO is even more so, given the distances involved. Apart from the danger of relying on complicated machinery for transferring the crew to its destination, the space environment itself is extremely harmful to human beings. Many of the problems encountered in human space travel deal with keeping the crew alive. Interplanetary space as well as the lunar and Martian surfaces are extremely hostile environments, including hard vacuum, extreme temperatures, space debris, zero or reduced gravity, as well as harmful radiation. It is this later aspect, the harmful radiation, that this case study will focus on as it constitutes the greatest uncertainty in respect to effects and mitigation. Mitigation efforts regarding vacuum, temperatures and debris are possible, based on proper spaceship and astronaut suit construction as well as effective operational design. The effects of reduced gravity have been extensively studied and countermeasures are in existence (Blaber et al. 2010). These countermeasures cannot eliminate the side effects of long duration space travel but can reduce them to the point that the crew remains operational for the duration of the mission. The issue of harmful radiation is rather more complex. There are currently no effective strategies for complete shielding from space radiation. Any human in space thus will be exposed, with exposure being relative to the duration and type of each mission.

---

[1] https://www.nasa.gov/specials/artemis-accords/index.html.

9.2.1   Space Radiation Physics

The main sources of radiation in space are galactic cosmic rays (GCRs) and solar particle events (SPEs). GCR are very energetic and thus highly penetrating. They are very difficult to attenuate and essentially cannot be stopped by shielding, since shield mass in space is limited. Spacecrafts cannot carry a heavy amount of shielding material (putting mass in orbit is very expensive), and a "weak" shield might in fact be worse than no shield at all, since a GCR will create a cascade of secondary particles of shield material that will saturate the insides of the spacecraft. It is thus preferable to let GCRs just pass through the human body.

SPEs include particles such as helium ions and other ions. SPEs originate at the Sun. These events occur sporadically with varying frequency. Frequency and intensity of SPEs are unpredictable, although they are related to the Solar 11-year cycle (solar minimum/maximum). Low energy SPE protons cannot penetrate spacecrafts or astronaut suits, but the high energy particles can, and thus contribute to astronaut radiation exposure. However, shielding (especially within a spacecraft) is effective against SPEs. Issues arise with astronauts outside the spacecraft (extravehicular activities) or exposed on the lunar or Martian surface, since when an SPE occurs, astronauts may not have time to seek protective shelter.

GCR flux can be modelled and expected exposure calculated. SPEs can be shielded against based on assumptions about intensity and frequency and planning of activities. Prediction of SPEs is not possible but advanced warning once one has occurred is feasible, albeit with a very small reaction timeframe.

9.2.2   Current Practises

Currently, space agencies have regulations that define radiation exposure standards that astronauts should not exceed. For example, NASA defines space permissible exposure limits (SPELs) for their astronauts which indicate that "astronauts shall not exceed 3% *risk of exposure-induced death* (REID) from cancer". The current NASA standard is adjusted for age and sex, which is not the case for all space agencies. The SPEL indicates an upper 95% confidence limit that the individual will die from cancer associated with the radiation exposure that the individual received while in space. In essence, out of 100 astronauts that have travelled in space, 3 might die from radiation related cancer. This is calculated for each astronaut, based on sex and age.

Radiation exposure dose equivalent unit in dosimetry is measured (in SI units) in sieverts (Sv). For exposure to small doses of ionising radiation, it is easier to use the millisievert (mSv). The current standards of the international space station partners can be seen in Table 9.1.

Table 9.1 Radiation exposure career limits for astronauts. ISS partner agencies. Adopted from NAS (2021)

Space agency	Career dose limit	Sex/age dependency
Canadian Space Agency	1000 mSv	No
European Space Agency	1000 mSv	No
Russian Federal Space Agency	1000 mSv	No
Japanese Aerospace Exploration Agency	3% REID	Yes Lower limit: 500 mSv (female, 27–30 years old) Upper limit:1000 mSv (male, >46 years old)
National Aeronautics and Space Administration	3% REID	Yes Lower limit:180 mSv (female, 30 years old) Upper limit: 700 mSv (male, 60 year old)

Table 9.2 Mission profile and duration with observed radiation dose (averaged). Adapted from NASA's space radiation FAQ[2]

Mission	Radiation dose
Space Shuttle 41-C (8 days, 460 km orbit)	5.59 mSv
Apollo 14 (9 days Lunar mission)	11.4 mSv
Skylab 4 (87 days, 473 km orbit)	178 mSv
ISS Mission (6 months, 353 km orbit)	160 mSv (Solar minimum)–80 mSv (Solar Maximum)
Average human on earth	~2 mSv per year from background radiation (location, lifestyle dependent)
Annual limit for workers dealing with radioactive material	50 mSv
Expected dose for average nuclear facility worker	1 mSv per year (adapted from ncr.gov[3])

To get an indication of how mission profiles affect radiation exposure, Table 9.2 summarises the radiation dose (average) for various mission types. Despite the difference in the type of radiation, 1 mSv of space radiation is roughly equivalent to receiving three chest X-rays.

Radiation doses are cumulative. Thus, under the current standards, a 30-year-old female NASA astronaut might be able to fly once or twice to the ISS before reaching her career limit, whereas a male astronaut can probably fly more times. For Russian, European or Canadian astronauts, longer or more missions can be undertaken. Note

[2] https://srag.jsc.nasa.gov/spaceradiation/faq/faq.cfm.

[3] Occupational Radiation Exposure at Commercial Nuclear Power Reactors and Other Facilities annual reports.

that older astronauts have higher exposure limits, as the overall impact on the rest of their lives is less than the impact on a younger astronaut.

9.2.3 Effects of Space Radiation on Human Health

Exposure to large doses of harmful radiation can signify increase risk for the development of cancer and non-cancer anomalies, such as leukaemia, circulatory diseases, vision impairing cataracts, cognitive and memory problems, potential heritable effects and infertility (Cucinotta and Durante 2006; Chylack et al. 2009; NRC 2006). The great degree of uncertainty about whether an astronaut will develop any of these health problems, especially cancer, makes it challenging to communicate these risks to astronauts, the public and policy makers. There are several sources of uncertainty.

As mentioned in the previous section, the average flux of GCR and solar activity can be simulated and modelled. However, SPEs are stochastic events, as there is no way to know exactly when and where an SPE will take place. Thus, it can be treated as a random occurrence, and therefore there is always a risk for a high energy event that exceeds the modelling parameters.

Another source of uncertainty is the actual effects of radiation on the human body. This might be surprising at first, given that radiation sources have been available for decades on Earth. Considering the effects of *long-term* exposure to radiation (rather than acute radiation exposure), however, showcases the difficulty of gathering data over a long period of time (decades) for large groups of exposed humans in order to conduct statistical studies and infer accurate risk rates.

Risk projections for cancer specific illnesses have largely been based on data from the Life Span Study (LSS) of the Japanese atomic bomb survivors. Additional data sources are being made available, such as studies of occupational radiation. Nevertheless, uncertainties remain regarding potential long-term effects (Chylack et al. 2009; NRC 2006).

9.2.4 Leaving Earth

The current space radiation exposure standards (see Table 9.1) were developed with short space missions in mind, planning for repeated missions (i.e. multiple stays in the ISS), where it was possible to return to Earth (and have access to health care there) within days. In venturing outside the Earth, to travel to the Moon and Mars, this will no longer be the case. In the case of travel to Mars, the round trip can take more than two years with the projected technology (for 2030+). The mission profile calls for a 6-month cruise, 18 months surface stay (waiting for Mars and Earth to re-align in their orbits and reduce necessary travel time) and 6 months travel back. Thus, once the mission has begun, an astronaut cannot decide that he or she no longer

Table 9.3 Mission profiles for future space exploration scenarios and expected radiation doses. Adopted from (Cucinotta and Durante 2006). Risk calculations can be found therein

Mission type	Effective dose (mSv) from GCR
Lunar Mission (180 Days)	170
Mars Orbit (600 days)	1030
Mars exploration (1000 days)	1070

wants to be part of it. This is quite different from what is typically found in terrestrial occupations that include radiation exposure. Terrestrial workers can choose to leave their job and thus end their exposure. Furthermore, the radiation environment outside Low Earth Orbit changes.

The most important factors that contribute to the heightened risk of radiation exposure for astronauts in Lunar or Mars exploration missions can thus be inferred from the above. Once outside the Earth's protective global magnetic field, which the Moon and Mars do not have (there are localised but not global magnetic fields), the flux of radiation (both GCR and SPEs in origin) increases. Additionally, the response window for energetic SPEs diminishes, as Solar observatories have to observe the event and a signal communicated to the astronauts needs to happen for them to take shelter. The further they are from Earth, the longer it will take for the message to be transmitted to them. In addition, the expected mission durations increase quite substantially, essentially placing future astronauts in a more hostile environment than they operate now, for much longer periods. Contrast Table 9.2 with expected radiation doses for future extra-terrestrial exploration missions (Table 9.3).

9.3 Ethical Space Exploration

The previous section highlights several issues regarding future space exploration destinations.

1. The effects of radiation will probably not have a technological mitigation measure in the envisaged timeframe for these countermeasures to be available. Thus, exposure to harmful radiation is a given for any mission.
2. Uncertainty still remains about the types of adverse effects that astronauts will incur due to long duration spaceflight. This makes it hard to accurately inform the crew on the impact of each mission on the participant's long-term health and quality of life.
3. For missions to Mars, termination of participation might not be an option. If the astronaut so chooses, he cannot just stop participating in the mission. The physical distances and planetary alignment might make it impossible to return to Earth, outside the planned window.
4. Given that exposure is cumulative, Lunar and Mars missions might necessitate inexperienced astronauts as crew (no previous exposure).

5. The current standards for astronaut lifetime radiation exposure do not actually allow participation in missions to Mars, as the nominal mission scenarios would exceed the allowable limits.

The points above ultimately create the situation that a future Mars mission will put the crew in harm's way, regarding career-received radiation, with increased risk of adverse health effects. This section will now describe the official (space agency) response and efforts to deal with this situation.

Spaceflight is an endeavour that brings benefits to many (society, scientists, future astronauts, etc.) but the risks are shared by a few (astronauts and their families), especially health risks. The astronaut corps can be considered an elite group of people, selected from a wide pool of willing candidates. Given the formation and training that the astronaut candidates receive once selected, it is difficult to claim that they are not aware of the risks for space flight and that they are not consenting to them.

The approach of NASA and other space agencies to address Mars as an exploration destination for astronauts is to offer a mission specific waiver for astronauts in such missions. Thus, explicitly informed consent will be needed for each member of a potential crew. As of today, only NASA allows for such a process, although other space agencies seem to agree with this approach.[4] It is highly probable that NASA will lead the way on this issue as the US has more mature plans for future space exploration. Thus, the US response to the problem will most probably define the responses of other agencies.

NASA has asked a committee of experts, brought together by the National Academies of Sciences, Engineering and Medicine (NAS), to review the current process for assessment and management of long-term risk with respect to cancer for crews (NAS 2021). The committee, which was comprised of experts in several related fields, such as radiation dosimetry, clinical oncology, biostatistics, physics, risk communication and management as well as former astronauts, offered recommendations to the agency. The full report also discusses NASA's plan to move to a different exposure limit standard, which will increase allowable career exposure limit that is common for all astronauts (male and female). The standard in question still remains more conservative that other space agencies with a unified approach (600 mSv for all, as opposed to 1000 mSv that is the standard for other agencies, as seen in Table 9.1). However, even with the new proposed standard, Mars missions will still require a waiver, and thus the situation as seen in the previous sections, remains similar.

It is of interest to note some of the recommendations made to NASA by the NAS committee (2021), regarding ethical issues.

Recommendation 2: *"In the near future, NASA should re-examine whether to use risk of exposure-induced death (REID) or other metrics, or a combination of metrics, in setting the dose-based space radiation health standard. NASA should conduct an*

---

[4] Regarding China, no data on astronaut exposure limits or waiver procedures were readily available so this section might not apply to Chinese practises.

independent analysis of the validity of 3% REID and make explicit the agency's justification for the metrics they choose."

The key element in the above recommendation is the need to make explicit the justification for the metrics to be used, regardless of the standards. This is sage advice and the foundation for creating trust in the standards. The main issue in the case of astronauts is that the current standards differentiate between male and female astronauts, but the proposed future standard is a common standard (based on a 35-year-old female) that, given the physiological differences, will allow more exposure to young, female astronauts but less exposure to older, male astronauts (which they could have been allowed with the older standard). As such, there is a trade-off between equality of opportunity for all versus restrictions imposed on a subgroup. Thus, the need for disclosure on the justification of choice, which will make explicit the argumentation for the change and present the ethical arguments that were evaluated against each other, which will help reassure the subgroup that might feel that their opportunity is being unfairly diminished, and that their position has been considered.

For missions regarding a waiver, it was recommended to follow the previous recommendations of a work on Health standards for spaceflight (IoM 2014), and to *"Adopt an Ethics-Based Decision Framework, NASA should apply the relevant ethics principles and fulfil the concomitant responsibilities through a three-level, ethics-based decision framework that examines (i) decisions about allowing risk to astronaut health and safety in excess of that permitted by health standards, (ii) decisions about undertaking specific missions, and (iii) decisions concerning individual astronaut participation and crew composition"* (IoM 2014, Recommendation 4).

It is understood that current exposure standards cannot apply for future missions to Mars (and some Moon missions). Thus, a waiver is the only way forward. The proposed, ethics-based decision framework, will then be used to decide who can join which mission. The three proposed levels of decision in the framework concern:

(i)   the decision that a waiver is indeed ethically acceptable, for which kind of missions and the criteria for the mission objectives and parameters for a waiver to be a possible option. This is necessary to minimise the use of a waiver and avoid a situation where all missions are indeed possible, given that a waiver can be granted.

(ii) The second decision level concerns each individual mission and whether it meets the criteria established in the previous level and thus a waiver is ethically acceptable. Finally,

(iii) the third decision level, which includes the crew composition for the selected mission. The objective here is to acquire *informed consent* and thus, it is necessary to provide as complete information as possible on flight risks, risk management plans and also the state of research knowledge that has informed the risks. The complete framework and decision points can be seen in the IoM report (2014, 145–150).

The way to communicate such risks to astronauts was also a main consideration in the more recent report (NAS 2021). The current paradigm is to use REID (Sect. 9.2.2) and distribution statistics based on age and gender. As an example (NAS, figure S-2), the risk associated with an effective dose of >600 mSv and thus above the NASA allowable limits, is indicated, highlighted red, as: High Risk—requires Agency Waiver—REID >2.27% mean (0.6, 7.8%) 95% CI for a 35-year-old female.

Even though astronauts are highly trained individuals, with advanced knowledge of risk statistics, it seems that even amongst astronauts the above type of communication is still confusing; effective dose as the main communicating tool would be preferred (NAS 2021, 14). It is interesting to note that it seems (based on discussions between active astronauts and the committee) that communication regarding reproductive health and possible issues from exposure might influence decisions in context for astronauts. The recommendations regarding risk communication to NASA were to:

- Assess and communicate risk at an individual level (rather than generic) for all astronauts
- Follow up the statistical presentation of risks with individualised discussion and answers to possible questions, in order to address questions from individual astronauts.
- Provide access to addition information as needed.
- Develop risk-based communication that is based on what astronauts want, how they process risk information and identify who and what are the most effective sources of information for them.

9.4   Conclusions

Transparency and full informed consent are critical in decision making regarding future exploration missions, even in the context of highly motivated individuals, such as the astronaut corps. It is highly unlikely that there will be no volunteers for a mission to Mars; the opposite is more likely. That, however, does not alleviate the ethical requirement of volunteers to have consented to be placed in such a situation.

There is another concern regarding future space exploration that has to do with the nascent era of commercial space flight. The year 2020 saw the first commercial crewed flight to the ISS, with the Space-X Demo 2 mission.[5] In early 2021, the same spacecraft, Dragon from SpaceX, carried, in addition to the US astronauts, one European and one Japanese astronaut to the ISS.[6] 2021 also saw the first suborbital flights from Virgin Galactic and Blue Origin, which were highly publicised as the respective CEOs were on board. However, both these flights were suborbital, as they did not achieve orbit, but rather flew close to the "edge of space", the Kármán line, an altitude of 100 km that defines the boundary between the beginning of space and Earth's atmosphere (this is an artificial boundary and does differ between nations. Blue Origin's New Shepherd vehicle flew above 100 km and Virgin Galactic's Unity

---

[5] https://www.nasa.gov/image-feature/demo-2-launching-into-history.

[6] https://www.lefigaro.fr/sciences/thomas-pesquet-a-ete-mis-sur-orbite-par-spacex-20210423.

22 flew below it).[7] Given the brevity of the suborbital flights (4–5 min of microgravity), the issues with exposure discussed in this article do not apply and thus suborbital space tourism is not considered at present.

Commercial spaceflight, and in future commercial space exploration, do need to be considered. There are discussions for commercial crew missions to the Moon and Mars as well, although currently, it is difficult to gauge their preparedness level. SpaceX does indicate future missions on its website to Moon and Mars with their Starship design (see for example: https://www.spacex.com/human-spaceflight/) but as of August 2021, there are not many details about these missions. Nevertheless, one can imagine that given the effects of radiation on the human body and that ill effects can manifest after several years or decades of someone exposed to radiation in space, it might be difficult for commercial companies to offer comprehensive informed consent information to potential astronauts, as they may not have the necessary data. Currently, only the national space agencies can dedicate resources to investigate the uncertainty regarding space radiation effects. Thus, space agency astronaut guidelines, standards and procedures may be adopted by potential commercial endeavours or at least be available as the "industry standard".

The conclusion from this case study is an extrapolation from the very specific group of people that constitute the astronaut corps. If candidates to be the first human to reach Mars or to walk on the Moon once again, still prefer fully informed consent procedures to be put in place, it is therefore evident that such a process should follow any decision regarding any group that is tasked with performing an action that will inherit some sort of risk. Policy makers, as representatives of society in such situations, need to ensure that society demonstrates its appreciation and support to the ones it asks to put themselves in harm's way, by ensuring that they do it knowing the full reasons and consequences of doing so. Thus, public agencies need to be constantly mindful of the ethical implications of their work, incorporate ethical decision making where relevant and ensure a continuous discursive engagement regarding the societal state of what is considered ethical.

References

Blaber, E., H. Marçal, and B.P. Burns. 2010. Bioastronautics: The influence of microgravity on astronaut health. *Astrobiology* 10 (5): 463–473. https://doi.org/10.1089/ast.2009.0415.

Chylack Jr., L. T., L. E. Peterson, A. H. Feiveson, M. L. Wear, F. K. Manuel, W. H. Tung, D. S. Hardy, L. J. Marak, and F. A. Cucinotta. 2009. NASA study of cataract in astronauts (NASCA). Report 1: Cross-sectional study of the relationship of exposure to space radiation and risk of lens opacity. *Radiation Research* 172(1): 10–20. https://doi.org/10.1667/RR1580.1.

Cucinotta, Francis A., and Marco Durante. 2006. Cancer risk from exposure to galactic cosmic rays: Implications for space exploration by human beings. *Lancet Oncology* 7 (5): 431–435. https://doi.org/10.1016/S1470-2045(06)70695-7.

---

[7] https://earthsky.org/human-world/the-billionaire-space-race-and-the-karman-line/.

IoM (Institute of Medicine). 2014. *Health standards for long duration and exploration space-flight: Ethics principles, responsibilities, and decision framework*. Washington, DC: The National Academies Press. https://doi.org/10.17226/18576.

NAS (National Academies of Sciences, Engineering, and Medicine). 2021. *Space radiation and astronaut health: Managing and communicating cancer risks*. Washington, DC: The National Academies Press.

NRC (National Research Council). 2006. *Health risks from exposure to low levels of ionizing radiation, BEIR VII Phase 2*. Washington, DC: The National Academies Press.

Chapter 10
Ethics Versus the Law: The Case of the Belfast Project

Helen Kara

Abstract This chapter offers a case study of the Belfast Project archive, set up by Boston College in the US to hold accounts of the conflict in Northern Ireland known as 'the Troubles'. People who provided information were given written guarantees that their own accounts, and indeed the Project itself, would be kept secret until after their deaths. However, the existence of the Project was made public by its own director while some participants were still alive. The chapter begins with a brief background to the Troubles and an explanation of the importance of archives. Then the history of the archive is outlined and analysed, and the lessons learned from the case are discussed. One key lesson is that unless or until there is legal recognition of researcher-participant privilege, it will not always be possible for research data to be kept secure both ethically and legally. In conclusion, we outline the potential role for archival evidence in policymaking, and provide evidence for the importance of trust in social co-operation. We point to ways in which policy can help to build and maintain this trust and so help to forestall and manage conflict.

Keywords Belfast Project · Boston College · Troubles · Northern Ireland · Ethics · Law · Case study · Violent conflict

10.1 Introduction

This chapter offers a case study of the Belfast Project, set up by Boston College in the US in the early twenty-first century. The Project's remit was to collect and store accounts of the late twentieth century conflict in Northern Ireland commonly known as 'the Troubles'. People who provided accounts for the Project were given written guarantees that not only their own accounts, but also the Project itself, would be kept secret until after their deaths. However, some years later, information about the Project was made public by the Project's own director while some of its participants were still alive, with complex and far-reaching consequences.

H. Kara (✉)
Independent Researcher, Uttoxeter, UK
e-mail: helen@weresearchit.co.uk

Researching violent conflicts inevitably raises difficult ethical issues (Brigden and Gohdes 2020). This chapter covers some of the ethical issues raised by the Belfast Project and, in so doing, explores the inherent tension between research ethics and legal ethics (Adams 2014).

10.2 Background

10.2.1 The Troubles

The Northern Ireland conflict of the late twentieth century, known as 'the Troubles', was a political and sectarian conflict over whether Northern Ireland should remain within the UK, or leave and form a united Ireland with the Irish Republic. The Troubles began in the late 1960s and ended around the late 1990s or early 2000s. It is difficult to date the conflict precisely, as there were several significant events and developments in the late 1960s, each of which could be held to be the start of the Troubles, and there is a similar picture in the late 1990s/early 2000s for the end of the Troubles (Fitzduff and O'Hagan 2009).

The Troubles is not an isolated conflict. In fact, as long ago as the early 1600 s, Scottish and English settlers colonised the north-east of Ireland, forcing the Irish people who lived there from their homelands (Fitzduff and O'Hagan 2009). This colonisation is known as the Ulster Plantation. The settlers were Protestant and had strong cultural ties with Scotland and England; the Irish people were Catholic and culturally Irish. The inequalities between these two sections of the population were never redressed and non-violent and violent conflicts have occurred regularly in Northern Ireland over the last four centuries (Fitzduff and O'Hagan 2009).

In 1801 the United Kingdom (UK) was formed. At that time the UK was made up of England, Scotland, Wales and the whole of Ireland. After the First World War there was an Irish war of independence which led to the formation of the Irish Free State, now known as the Republic of Ireland. Northern Ireland as it exists today was formed by legislation passed in 1921 partitioning the island of Ireland (Fitzduff and O'Hagan 2009). This placed the counties of Antrim, Armagh, Down, Fermanagh, Londonderry and Tyrone in Northern Ireland, and the other 26 counties in the South.

The name 'Londonderry' is contested, with most of those supporting the Union favouring the name Londonderry, while most Irish nationalists prefer Derry. This is just one example of the polarisation of society in Northern Ireland; at a more macro level, 'peace walls' were built during the Troubles along streets in several towns and cities to keep nationalists and unionists apart in an effort to reduce violence (McGrade 2017).

In the early 1960s a number of initiatives were developed in Northern Ireland to combat discrimination against Catholics. By 1967 these had cohered into a civil rights movement with the formation of the Northern Ireland Civil Rights Association (NICRA) which aimed to secure the rights of all citizens, regardless of their religious or political affiliations, through public protests on the streets (McKenna undated). However, unionists saw NICRA as being a republican, not an egalitarian, organisation, and accused it of working to undermine the state of Northern Ireland. Civil unrest reached a peak in summer 1969 and after the 'battle of the Bogside', the name given to three days of violent confrontation between Catholic residents and Northern Irish police in Derry/Londonderry, resulting in the British Government deploying British troops to keep the peace on the streets of Northern Ireland, where they remained until the early twenty-first century. In 1972 the civil rights movement ended, and NICRA was disbanded when London suspended the Northern Ireland parliament and took control of the region from Westminster.

Thousands of people were killed in the Troubles and tens of thousands were injured. Those who were killed included 1,785 civilians, more than half of whom were killed by loyalist paramilitaries, and over 1,100 British soldiers, most of whom were killed by republican paramilitaries (Sutton undated). Although peace then prevailed for the most part for over 20 years, the post-Brexit uprisings demonstrated that feelings on the issues could still be very strong.

10.2.2 Archives

An archive is a collection of documents or other records of historical interest, and/or the place where such a collection or collections are stored. This storage may be in digital or bricks-and-mortar spaces. Archives are usually seen as neutral, inactive resources which people can use at will for academic, cultural, or recreational purposes. However, archives are not value-free, and not all archives are accessible to everyone. Archives can also be seen as a form of power, an attempt to control the past by privileging some stories and marginalising others (Schwartz and Cook 2002), and/or by placing restrictions on who can use, and when and how they can have access to, the archival material. Archives 'are not passive storehouses of old stuff, but active sites where social power is negotiated, contested, confirmed' (Schwartz and Cook 2002, 1).

Archives are often associated with institutions. Institutional archives usually have policies to govern their operation. However, these policies vary a great deal between different institutions (Wood et al. 2014). There are no overarching rules or guidelines governing the policies of an institutional archive so, in essence, an institution can write its own policy.

Archivists know that in post-conflict situations, 'documenting or disclosing the provenance of materials may put those who created, collected or provided those materials at considerable risk' (Wood et al. 2014, 412–3). There is also risk that the materials, so carefully created, collected or provided, may be destroyed or relocated and so lost to history.

Collections of records that document any violent and systematic abuse of power may be known as 'human rights archives' (Caswell 2014, 208). These can include stories recorded by survivors of a human rights crisis. Creating, preserving, and using records documenting human rights crises, such as the Troubles, is a process fraught with political, ethical, legal and cultural challenges (Caswell 2014).

10.3   The Case Study

In 2001, the Burns Library of Boston College in the US set up an oral history archive focusing on the Troubles. The archive was known as the Belfast Project. The intention was to include perspectives of those on both sides of the conflict, to ensure accurate records that could not be lost or distorted by history. This was important because there was, and is, a high level of disagreement between loyalists and republicans about what constitutes 'truth' and 'facts' about the Troubles and related issues (Inckle 2015). The Project director was Ed Moloney, who had a background as an Irish journalist covering the Troubles, and in 1999 had fought and won a court case against a court order he had received to hand over some journalistic interview notes of interest to UK anti-terrorist authorities (Palys and Lowman 2012).

Moloney recruited insider researchers—two academics who were also convicted ex-paramilitaries, one Loyalist and one Republican—to conduct extended interviews with participants from their own side of the conflict (Inckle 2015). These were research interviews rather than journalistic interviews. The 'Agreement between the Trustees of Boston College and Edward Moloney, Project Director, to Interview Members of Irish Republican Paramilitary Organizations and Provisional Sinn Fein Regarding their Role in the "Troubles"' states that interviews are to be documented on audio or video tape and transcribed (Belfast Project Agreement 2001). Transcripts would be deposited in the archive, together with signed statements of authenticity, under an alphanumeric code for anonymity. The key providing the link between codes and names would be kept in Boston and could only be seen by the Project director and the librarian who managed the archive. These protections were put in place because the interviews would inevitably include secret information, such as accounts of criminal activities including bombings and murders, and that information would be dangerous for participants and others if it became public (Inckle 2015). Over the next nine years, the interviewers conducted over 200 interviews which were placed in the archive.

Boston College gave the researchers 'Agreement for Donation' forms for participants to sign, guaranteeing that the information they provided would be kept safely within the archive until after their death. Even so, pseudonyms were used and, as we have seen, careful processes to protect participants' anonymity were put in place (Cardenas 2019). Furthermore, the whole Belfast Project was to be kept secret, with both interviewer and interviewee required to sign an agreement stating that neither would tell anyone else about the Project without permission from Boston College. The intention here was to ensure that participants felt able to give complete and truthful accounts of their experiences in the Troubles (Inckle 2015). The Belfast Project Agreement, signed by Ed Moloney in 2001, said 'Each interviewee is to be given a contract guaranteeing to the extent that American law allows the conditions of the interview and the conditions of its deposit…' but this potential limitation was not communicated to participants (Palys and Lowman 2012). In practice, nobody working on the Project, in the US or in Northern Ireland, had any idea that they could be forced to make interview transcripts or recordings available to a third party while interviewees were still alive (Breen-Smyth 2019).

In 2010 Ed Moloney published *Voices From The Grave*, a book based on interviews with two of the Project's participants, loyalist David Ervine who had died in 2007 and republican Brendan Hughes who had died in 2008. The book was accompanied by a TV documentary with the same name. The Irish media became interested, which brought the Project to the attention of the UK legal authorities, who learned that the archive might contain evidence to help them clear up unsolved murders from the conflict. The UK Government asked the US Attorney General to subpoena Boston College to make them hand over all material related to two of the interviews, and the subpoenas were delivered in May 2011 (Palys and Lowman 2012). Delivery of one interview was straightforward because the participant had died. The other participant was still alive and, after much legal argument, Boston College handed over the material to the court for a judge to read and make the final decision. After due consideration the judge decided to release the material to the UK Government.

This action by Boston College did not contravene the Agreement the College signed with Ed Moloney, but did contravene the guarantee of protection given to participants on the 'Agreement for Donation' forms. Staff of Boston College argued that they had only guaranteed anonymity within the limits of the US legal system, not internationally, and so had to be bound by the judge's decision. The action of Boston College had terrifying consequences for members of the Project team, some of whom feared for their lives while others were advised not to travel to Northern Ireland because the risk was too high (Inckle 2015).

Ed Moloney feared further subpoenas and suggested moving the archive to the Republic of Ireland, but Boston College disagreed. In August 2011 a second set of subpoenas were delivered to Boston College, this time asking for 'any and all… information' contained in the archive about an unsolved murder (Cullen 2011). More legal argument ensued, with Ed Moloney and one of the interviewers getting involved in filing motions and swearing affidavits to try to protect the participants. This time Boston College handed over half of the archive to the court for a judge to read and make the final decision. In February 2012 the American Sociological Association, and members of the Boston College Chapter of the American Association of University Professors, made public statements of support for the researchers. However, the judge gave the UK police access to material deemed to be relevant to criminal inquiries (Breen-Smyth 2019).

While it was good news for the UK criminal justice system, this had major consequences for several republicans and loyalists who had participated, or been named, in the interviews. In March 2014, the republican former IRA leader, Ivor Bell, was arrested and charged with soliciting the murder of Jean McConville in 1972. In April 2014, the republican Sinn Féin leader Gerry Adams was taken in for questioning and was released several days later without charge. Bobby Storey, another Sinn Féin leader, was arrested in December 2014 and later released without charge. In June

2016, the loyalist former Ulster Volunteer Force and Red Hand Commando member 'Winkie' Rea was charged with 19 offences including aiding and abetting murder and conspiracy to murder. All of these actions were based on evidence from the Belfast Project (Breen-Smyth 2019).

In May 2014, Boston College offered to return interviews to their originators on request. But this was too little, too late, and the legal processes continued. In July 2016 it was announced that Ivor Bell would stand trial, charged with 'encouraging persons to murder Mrs McConville and endeavouring to persuade persons to murder her' (BBC 2019). However, Bell had developed vascular dementia so was deemed unfit to stand trial. This led to a legal process known as 'a trial of the facts', in which the truth of the allegations against a defendant is examined rather than the defendant's guilt or innocence of the crime with which they have been charged. As a result of this process, the judge, Mr Justice O'Hara, ruled that the evidence provided by the recordings was unreliable. In particular, the judge ruled that the researcher had asked leading questions, and that the promise of confidentiality, while designed to promote truth-telling, could equally have given the interviewee freedom to tell lies, distort the truth, or mislead the researcher (McKeown 2019). As a result, in October 2019 Ivor Bell was acquitted of involvement in the murder of Jean McConville.

10.4   Analysis

It is very difficult for researchers or participants to assess all the potential risks that may arise from doing or taking part in research. People are generally poor judges of risk, for a range of reasons such as having inaccurate or incomplete information, biases including optimism bias or availability bias, and the important role of context. Also, risk is particularly difficult to perceive when it is in the future because of the increased levels of uncertainty which mean the past is not always a trustworthy guide. Power dynamics, in particular, can change in unexpected ways, with potentially harmful implications for research participants and researchers (Parkinson and Wood 2015; Brigden and Gohdes 2020). Also, advances in technology can cause inaccessible or private information to become accessible (Bridgen and Gohdes 2020). As the case of the Belfast Project shows, there is even uncertainty about whether research institutions will keep their promises when facing external pressure (Thaler 2021). This level of uncertainty seriously compromises the principle of informed consent because it is not possible fully to inform someone about the risks they would be taking if they participate in research (Parkinson and Wood 2015). And it is not only researchers and participants who may be endangered by research, but also the 'unintended research participants' (Bridgen and Gohdes 2020, 256) or 'non-consenting others' (Mannay 2016, 123) who may be involved by being mentioned by participants without their knowledge or simply by having a stake in the research topic, such as by being on one side or the other in a sectarian conflict like the Troubles.

Some human rights archives 'can play a key role in helping societies deal with painful pasts and build peaceful futures' (Caswell 2014, 209). The Belfast Project had the opposite effect. The actions listed above, taken as a result of the Belfast Project, are only those we know about. The exposure of the Belfast Project will, if nothing else, have caused alarm and fear, stress and anxiety to surviving participants and their families and friends. Making any data from this kind of research available to people outside the research team can lead to retaliation and great damage to individuals and communities (Parkinson and Wood 2015). Also, this kind of case damages research as a whole, with reputational damage to researchers whether or not they were involved with the Belfast Project itself, and decreased willingness of potential participants to take part in future research. The twenty-first century has seen increasing calls for archives to take an active role in pursuing human rights and social justice (Wood et al. 2014). This case study functions as a cautionary tale within the ongoing conversations around the possibilities and challenges of working in this way (ibid).

Some might argue that the ethical problems in this case are linked to the specific research method used, i.e. interviewing, or—more broadly—that these kinds of ethical problems are inherent in qualitative research. However, it is clear from other research that the 'politics of information' affects research into political violence that uses a wide range of methods, from ethnographic participant observation to quantitative and digital research (Bridgen and Gohdes 2020). Also, the problems created by the Belfast Project are not specific to oral history research. Regardless of the research method used, doing research with people who have been involved in violence can create short-term and long-term risks for both participants and the 'non-consenting others' (Mannay 2016, 123) named by participants. Giving people access to a research dataset, such as that contained in the Belfast Project archive, 'can bring to attention previously hidden connections, relationships, histories, and contexts that risk having harmful personal or political effects for research participants' (Bridgen and Gohdes 2020, 257). Furthermore, 'Entire communities might suffer "collateral damage" from research that makes sensitive information visible to a new audience' (Brigden and Gohdes 2020, 256).

One of the reasons given by Mr Justice O'Hara, the judge in Ivor Bell's 'trial of the facts', for ruling that the evidence was unreliable, was that the researcher had asked leading questions. Yet the Belfast Project researchers were recruited specifically from each side of the Troubles, to interview people from their own side. This makes sense because to gather information from people who are implicated in violent conflict, a researcher would need to demonstrate understanding of their participants' perspective on that conflict (Thaler 2021) and to be trusted, at least to some extent, by those participants. In this context, in the course of a qualitative interview which is in fact a conversation and where both parties to the dialogue know they share a perspective, some leading questions seem almost inevitable. Even if there were no leading questions, it is virtually impossible to exclude the influence of a researcher's own standpoint from data gathering (Thaler 2021), particularly when the researcher's standpoint is explicitly aligned with participants' standpoints. In this kind of research, data is not collected from participants by interviewers, it is constructed by participants and interviewers together. And other factors could render such 'evidence' as unreliable in legal terms, such as retrospective bias which inevitably affects the views and interpretations of participants and researchers when discussing events of the past (Thaler 2021). Yet for researchers, social commentators, historians and others, this kind of evidence is vital.

Research into violent conflict is suffused with power at macro and micro levels. Violent conflict itself is a display of power, often in response to other displays of power. Then there is the balance of power between researchers and participants, each of whom has the power to tell the truth or to lie, to keep or break promises. Wood et al. (2014, 401) assert that 'When power is denied, overlooked, or unchallenged, it is misleading at best and dangerous at worst. Power recognized becomes power that can be questioned, made accountable, and opened to transparent dialogue and enriched understanding'. But when legal or state power comes into play, this is not necessarily the case. Though those powers may be contested, it may not be possible—at least in the short term—to question them or to demand accountability.

Archives in general have been described as sites of power contestation, though this is usually more covert than in the case of the Belfast Project. Expressions of political and social power within and through archives are usually held to relate to who makes and uses archival records, and why (O'Toole 2002, 45). In the case of the Belfast Project the power contestation is more overt, with confidentiality and secrecy promised by researchers being breached, leading to legal tussles over access to confidential archival materials, and the release of some of those materials with dramatic consequences for both researchers and participants.

10.5 Lessons Learned

Violent conflict is a pressing social problem which often leaves an unwelcome legacy (Crooke 2010). This means conflict can recur after prolonged periods of calm, as shown by the Brexit-related uprisings in Northern Ireland in the spring of 2021 after 20 years of relative peace in the region. Research into the causes and consequences of violent conflict is essential for understanding how such conflict can be prevented or resolved (Thaler 2021). That research needs to be conducted with extreme care, and no promises should be made that will not be kept. Yet researchers also need to recognise that they may not always be able to safeguard the data they gather, though they should always make every effort to do so.

Truth and facts are not singular and identifiable but multiple and contested. This is the basis on which Boston College set up its archive, and this also plays out in the tussle between research ethics and legal ethics in this case. The criminal justice system is not the only mechanism that can put pressure on researchers to release confidential data. Academic journal publishers, editors, and peer reviewers have also done so (Parkinson and Wood 2015). Unless or until there is legal recognition of researcher-participant privilege, it will not always be possible for research data to be kept secure both ethically and legally.

The Belfast Project worked, initially, because Boston College and the Project staff created conditions in which trust could be established and built, and participants trusted the Project and the College—or, at least, the researcher they spoke with who was explicitly on their side. It is a testament to the Project that this trust was maintained even though they were gathering data from both sides of the conflict, when so much mistrust has built up between loyalists and republicans over many decades. Then, when the Project's existence was made public, contravening the conditions in which that trust existed, the trust broke down. The consequent reputational damage to Boston College, Belfast Project staff, and research, researchers and research institutions more generally, means the mistrust generated by the Project's breach of confidentiality is much more widespread than the trust built up by the Project before that breach. Reputations are slow to establish and grow, and quick to damage or destroy.

Kahryn Hughes and Anna Tarrant offer a useful summary of the implications of this case:

> At its simplest, the case of the Belfast Project established that, despite assurances to the contrary, the safeguarding and confidentiality of archived data is not necessarily always possible, or it might only be possible for certain sorts of data at given historical moments, regardless of the contractual agreements in place at the time consent is given or sought for archiving. Legal-political changes have the power to destabilise such agreements or contracts; and thus assurances given by organisations such as universities, or individuals such as researchers, cannot be understood as enduring for all time. The [Belfast Project] case is an extreme example that reflects the highly charged character of those particular data. Most interview data would not provoke international political interest and risk of this sort. Nevertheless, it is a useful example to underscore the changing and potentially fragile contexts through which data may pass, and the limits of researcher control and protection of them. (Hughes and Tarrant 2020, 45)

10.6   Implications and Recommendations for Efers

This case shows that, far from being inert resources, archives can 'engage in powerful public policy debates' (Schwartz and Cook 2002, 2). This is one reason why it is useful for policymakers to know about and understand archives. Another is that archives can provide a useful resource for policymakers. We know that policymakers use a variety of sources of evidence in their work, such as research evidence, theoretical evidence (ideas, concepts, models), expert advice, political and professional knowledge, and experiential evidence or testimony (Glasby 2011; Nutley et al. 2012; Sohn 2018; Bache 2019). There is also a role here for archival evidence. Someone making policy to help with conflict management might have found the Boston College archive to be a very useful resource.

In one sense, the case of the Belfast Project shows what can happen when policies come into conflict. In this case the Boston College policy on confidentiality for Belfast Project participants came into conflict with the criminal justice system policy of working to bring offenders to justice. Policy conflict is a complex arena with varying levels of intensity and action, affected by the different attributes and cognitive and behavioural characteristics of individual policy actors (Weible and Heikkila 2017). But put simply, when policies come into conflict, the people who operate those policies also come into conflict, each group trying to gain the upper hand. In the case of the Belfast Project, legal ethical policy won out over research ethical policy. However, there is no clear policy hierarchy at national or international level (though such a hierarchy may exist at institutional level), so it is possible that on another occasion, if operated differently, research ethical policy could prevail. And we know that policy conflicts can lead to new policies (Weible and Heikkila 2017). Perhaps this case will ultimately lead to more robust policies around researchers' rights to confidentiality, such as those which exist for journalists (Adams 2014). Some will argue that the requirements of the criminal justice system should take precedence over the ethics of research. However, researchers need to do everything they can to ensure the welfare of their participants, even when those participants are implicated in violent conflict, and this requirement should be supported by well-made policies.

The workings of violent conflicts are invisible to most people, as are the workings of researchers, and the workings of the state including the making of policy (Bridgen and Gohdes 2020, 263). Yet one factor linking violent conflicts, research, and policy-making is trust. Trust is often seen as an attribute of individuals, but it may be more useful to consider it as a resource which is essential for co-operation in complex societies (Cairney and Wellstead 2019). Of course, individuals base actions on 'trust calculations', but these inevitably exist within, and are influenced by, a wider context (Cairney and Wellstead 2019, 5). In essence, trust helps us to reduce uncertainty and get things done. When trust breaks down, we often turn to the law. Clearly the law has a vital role to play in our societies, but it is not perfect, and it can be a very blunt instrument. Policy can help to sharpen its edge.

Policymakers need to consider cases such as the Belfast Project when making policy about the management. storage and sharing of sensitive information. Flexibility within such policy is essential because of the evident level of uncertainty involved in gathering and storing information. It is clear that compelling researchers to share information can cause real harm to individual participants and their communities, and to researchers themselves. Managing uncertainty requires continual negotiation, adaptation, and improvisation, and scope for these should be built into any relevant policy.

These ethical dangers are not unique to cases involving primary data. Even if information about violent conflict is publicly available, using it as secondary data for research may bring it to more people's attention which could lead to 'new political incentives for retaliation against participants' (Bridgen and Gohdes 2020, 257). This can lead to reputational damage, loss of social status, ostracization and even more violence. Yet in order to make policy about violent conflict, policymakers need access to relevant findings from good quality ethical research. When legal or other requirements take precedence over research ethics, research is compromised, and findings which could be invaluable to the next generation of policymakers may not exist.

References

Adams, Katherine. 2014. The tension between research ethics and legal ethics: Using journalist's privilege state statutes as model for proposed researcher's privilege. *Georgetown Journal of Legal Ethics* 27 (3): 335–358.

Bache, Ian. 2019. How does evidence matter? Understanding 'what works' for wellbeing. *Social Indicators Research* 142: 1153–1173. https://doi.org/10.1007/s11205-018-1941-0.

BBC. 2019. Boston tapes: Q&A on secret Troubles confessions. https://www.bbc.co.uk/news/uk-northern-ireland-27238797. Accessed 7 Sep 2021.

Belfast Project Agreement. 2001. http://bostoncollegesubpoena.wordpress.com/exhibits/respondent-moloney-agreement/. Accessed 22 Jun 2021.

Breen-Smyth, Marie. 2019. Interviewing combatants: Lessons from the Boston College Case. *Contemporary Social Science* 15 (2): 258–274.

Brigden, Noelle K., and Anita R. Gohdes. 2020. The politics of data access in studying violence across methodological boundaries: What we can learn from each other? *International Studies Review* 22: 250–267. https://doi.org/10.1093/isr/viaa017.

Brigden, N., and A. Gohdes. 2020. The politics of data access in studying violence across methodological boundaries: What we can learn from each other? *International Studies Review* 22: 250–267. https://doi.org/10.1093/isr/viaa017

Cairney, Paul, and Adam Wellstead. 2019. The role of trust in policymaking. In *Paper to international conference on public policy*, Montreal, may. https://paulcairney.files.wordpress.com/2020/03/cairney-wellstead-icpp-trust-14.6. Accessed 13 Apr 2021.

Caswell, Michelle. 2014. Defining human rights archives: Introduction to the special double issue on archives and human rights. *Archival Science* 14: 207–213. https://doi.org/10.1007/s10502-014-9226-0.

Cardenas, Anne. 2019. Lessons from the Belfast Project. May 24. http://oralhistory.columbia.edu/blog-posts/lessons-from-the-belfast-project. Accessed 22 Apr 2021.

Crooke, Elizabeth. 2010. The politics of community heritage: Motivations, authority and control. *International Journal of Heritage Studies* 16 (1–2): 16–29.

Fitzduff, Mari, and Liam O'Hagan. 2009. The Northern Ireland Troubles: INCORE background paper. https://cain.ulster.ac.uk/othelem/incorepaper09.htm. Accessed 23 Jun 2021.

Flynn, Danny, and Scott Baker. 2019. BC Belfast Project case ends in acquittal. *The heights*, October 28. https://www.bcheights.com/2019/10/28/belfast/. Accessed 22 Apr 2021.

Glasby, Jon. 2011. From evidence-based to knowledge-based policy and practice. In *Evidence, policy and practice: Critical perspectives in health and social care*, ed. Jon Glasby, 85–98. Bristol: Policy Press.

Hughes, Kahryn, and Anna Tarrant. 2020. The ethics of qualitative secondary analysis. In *Qualitative secondary analysis*, ed. Kahryn Hughes and Anna Tarrant, 37–58. London: SAGE.

Inckle, Kay. 2015. Promises, promises: Lessons in research ethics from the Belfast Project and 'The Rape Tape' case. *Sociological Research Online* 20 (1): 59–71.

Mannay, Dawn. 2016. *Visual, narrative and creative research methods: Application, reflection and ethics*. Abingdon: Routledge.

McGrade, Niall. 2017. The story behind Northern Ireland's peace walls. https://theculturetrip.com/europe/united-kingdom/northern-ireland/articles/the-story-behind-northern-irelands-peace-walls/. Accessed 9 Sep 2021.

McKenna, Fionnula. Undated. "We Shall Overcome"… The history of the struggle for civil rights in Northern Ireland 1968–1978 by NICRA (1978). https://cain.ulster.ac.uk/events/crights/nicra/nicra781.htm. Accessed 7 Sep 2021.

McKeown, Lesley-Anne. 2019. The Troubles: former IRA man Ivor Bell cleared of Jean McConville charges. https://www.bbc.co.uk/news/uk-northern-ireland-50044269. Accessed 7 Sep 2021.

Nutley, Sandra Margaret, Alison Elizabeth Powell, and Huw Davies. 2012. What counts as good evidence? Provocation paper for the Alliance for Useful Evidence.

O'Toole, James M. 2002. Cortes's notary: The symbolic power of records. *Archival Science* 2: 45–61.

Palys, Ted, and John Lowman. 2012. Defending research confidentiality "to the extent the law allows:" Lessons from the Boston College subpoenas. *Journal of Academic Ethics* 10 (4): 271–297.

Parkinson, Sarah Elizabeth, and Elisabeth Jean Wood. 2015. Transparency in intensive research on violence: Ethical dilemmas and unforeseen consequences. *Qualitative & Multi-Method Research* 13 (1): 22–27. https://doi.org/10.5281/zenodo.893081.

Schwartz, Joan M., and Terry Cook. 2002. Archives, records, and power: The making of modern memory. *Archival Science* 2: 1–19.

Sohn, Jacqueline. 2018. Navigating the politics of evidence-informed policymaking: Strategies of influential policy actors in Ontario. *Palgrave Communications* 4: 49. https://doi.org/10.1057/s41599-018-0098-4.

Sutton, Malcolm. Undated. Sutton index of deaths. https://cain.ulster.ac.uk/sutton/index.html. Accessed 7 Sep 2021.

Thaler, Kai M. 2021. Reflexivity and temporality in researching violent settings: Problems with the replicability and transparency regime. *Geopolitics* 26 (1): 18–44. https://doi.org/10.1080/14650045.2019.1643721.

Weible, Christopher M., and Tanya Heikkila. 2017. Policy conflict framework. *Policy Science* 50: 23–40. https://doi.org/10.1007/s11077-017-9280-6.

Wood, Stacy, Kathy Carbone, Marika Cifor, Anne Gilliland, and Ricardo Punzalan. 2014. Mobilizing records: Re-framing archival description to support human rights. *Archival Science* 14: 397–419. https://doi.org/10.1007/s10502-014-9233-1.

https://archive.boston.com/news/local/massachusetts/articles/2011/06/09/bc_asks_for_ira_project_secrecy/?page=full

Chapter 11
Research and the Ethics of Urban Exploration and Criminal Trespass

Mark Israel

Abstract Bradley Garrett, an urban ethnographer, took part in exploration of British urban space that involved trespass onto land owned by the public transport authority. Garrett argued that it was 'deeply problematic' to block research on people simply because they lived close to 'legal boundaries'. He also argued that participant observation with such groups might entail breaking the law. In 2012, Garrett and eight participants were arrested and charged with conspiracy to commit criminal damage and the prosecution based its case on research notes seized from Garrett. The case ended with Garrett receiving a conditional discharge. This chapter uses this 'urban explorer' case study to explore the justifications that might exist for undertaking covert research, for researchers breaking the law or for doing harm to participants and other interested parties, the ethics of autoethnography, the dangers of romanticising the subject of research, and the difficulties of negotiating multiple roles as researcher, urban explorer, political activist, journalist and filmmaker.

Keywords Ethnography · Covert research · Crime · Autoethnography · Maleficence · Research ethics

11.1 Introduction

In August 2012 Bradley Garrett, an urban ethnographer, was arrested at Heathrow airport (Garrett 2014b). Four years earlier he had started doctoral research on 'urban explorers' or 'place hackers' in London and elsewhere. Underground tube stations proved to be particularly attractive for the research and in due course the British Transport Police (BTP) took note. Following his arrest, the BTP seized field notes and related research materials. Garrett and eight of his research participants were subsequently charged with 'conspiracy to commit criminal damage'—a charge that carries a ten-year prison sentence. The BTP also alleged that the amount of material they had collected from Garrett's home indicated he must have been the instigator

M. Israel (✉)
Senior Consultant, Australasian Human Research Ethics Consultancy Services, School of Social Sciences, University of Western Australia, Perth, WA, Australia
e-mail: mark.israel@ahrecs.com

© The Author(s) 2022
D. O'Mathúna and R. Iphofen (eds.), *Ethics, Integrity and Policymaking*, Research Ethics Forum 9, https://doi.org/10.1007/978-3-031-15746-2_11

of the crimes of 'trespass' and of the 'criminal damage' entailed in gaining access to the sites (Booth 2014).

Bradley Garrett's exploration of British urban space which involved trespass onto land owned by the public transport authority raised several concerns for social research. The prosecution argued Garrett's law-breaking was both unethical and unnecessary since he could have completed the work legally. They might also have pointed to the possibility that repeated trespass would have required the authority to spend more on security, a cost that would have been passed on to passengers. In turn, the defence drew on a range of experts (including members of the British Society of Criminology and the American Society of Criminology). Jeff Ferrell, in particular, indicated that if ethnography were to be 'deep and full' it might well require engagement in interactions and situation that are illegal (Ferrell et al. 2015). Garrett himself argued that it was 'deeply problematic' to block research by people simply because they lived close to 'legal boundaries'. He also noted that participant observation with such groups might involve breaking the law. The case ended with Garrett (2014b) receiving a conditional discharge. One might interpret the result as signifying successful defence of the principles of ethnography and the fact that research can sometimes take people beyond the boundaries of the law. A more prosaic and realistic interpretation might be that Garrett acknowledged trespass and very limited criminal damage but was not found guilty of conspiracy to commit criminal damage.

Public and private discussions about this case have been partly structured around an understandable desire both by Garrett and by those who wrote in support of him to guard against the threat of significant criminal sanctions being imposed. In that context, criticism of Garrett is easily interpreted as a threat to his wellbeing and even as a threat to specific kinds of research. In addition, as Robert Dingwall remarked in 1980, most researchers remain 'naturally reluctant to shop one another and ethical debate is stifled by a silent recognition that the next time one could be the target oneself' (Dingwall 1980, 882).

This study is not concerned with reaching a conclusion on the merits and faults of Garrett's specific activities. It is a complex and heated case. Instead, it uses the case as an entry point to some of the debates about research ethics that exist within ethnography, particularly as practiced in the disciplines of anthropology, sociology, geography and criminology.

In particular, it will explore the justifications that might exist for undertaking covert research, for researchers breaking the law or for doing harm to participants and other interested parties, the ethics of autoethnography, the dangers of romanticising the subject of research, and the difficulties of negotiating multiple roles.

11.2 What Ethnographers Do

Ethnography generally entails ethnographers taking part in the daily lives of a particular group of people over a lengthy period, watching, listening and asking questions about what they encounter. As a term, ethnography is losing some of its precision and is being used to cover an increasing range of data-gathering activities (Becker 2017)—while ethnography is often grounded in participant observation, it may involve informal conversation, interviews, group discussions, documentary analysis and an examination of other material objects including digital photography and video. The orientation is generally exploratory. Data collection tends to be unstructured and analytical categories grow from the data rather than being imposed from a pre-existing framework.

Garrett's work was an analysis of recreational trespass by groups of people who spend their leisure time exploring off-limits, closed off areas of our cities, including 'derelict industrial sites, closed mental hospitals, abandoned military installations, sewer and drain networks, transportation and utility tunnels, shuttered businesses, foreclosed estates, mines, construction sites, cranes, bridges and bunkers…' (Garrett 2014a, 1). As the list suggests, the incursions included 'infiltration' of 'live' sites currently in use. Garrett spent over three years living and working with over 100 participants, eventually focussing on approximately 24 members of a more active group called the London Consolidation Crew, a group within which he came to take a leadership role.

11.3   Covert Research

The default position in most research ethics guidelines is that research participants should consent to their involvement in research. The regulation of consent could operate in such a way that it protects the interests of vulnerable groups from harmful research carried out by government agencies. Alternatively, it could protect powerful agencies from scrutiny by independent researchers by robbing researchers of one of their more powerful methodologies, covert research. Deception could compromise both the informed and voluntary nature of consent, but some researchers have argued consent need not be obtained where any harm caused by lack of consent might be outweighed by the public benefit obtained, and I shall return to this later on. In addition, it might be impossible to gain access to some participants if other people were not deceived. Without covert research, Pearson (2009) argued, some aspects of society, including harms and injustices will remain 'hidden or misunderstood' (2009, 252) and the images that powerful groups wish to project may go unchallenged.

The European Commission's (2010) draft Guidance Note for social science researchers counselled against allowing powerful figures or organizations the right to withdraw or withhold consent for fear of leaving social scientists 'without even the most basic rights to make enquiries [held] by other social groups, such as investigative journalists, or even ordinary citizens who might confront such figures at public meetings' (2010, 11). The 2009 Finnish guidelines were explicit in relation to studying more powerful groups: 'As a matter of principle, studies on the use of power should be allowed without the consent of those in power' (National Advisory Board on Research Ethics 2009, s1.5). However, the value of covert research may be broader than 'studying up'. At one time, the significance of covert studies was identified in the United Kingdom by the Economic and Social Research Council in its 2015 Framework for Research Ethics in exceptional circumstances 'if important issues are being addressed and if matters of social significance which cannot be uncovered in other ways are likely to be discovered' (2015, 30). The question of what might make something socially significant and how this is to be assessed was left unclear and, without better guidance, human research ethics committees might have been vulnerable to political and institutional pressure on this matter.

Covert research may be a matter of degree. By the very nature of their activity, many ethnographers cannot seek to obtain consent from all the people with whom they interact, on every occasion. There can be no 'Danger: Ethnographer Present' sign that would make every person passing through a location aware that a researcher might be present. This might be the case because an ethnographer is observing someone's activities in a public location where the presence of other people is incidental to the focus of the study, because revealing their role might disrupt multiple social interactions or endanger the key research participant (Fountain 1993), or because over time the ethnographer becomes a taken-for-granted part of the setting whose reason for being there is no longer clearly remembered by others.

Garrett's research was not covert in any absolute sense—other urban explorers were aware that he was a doctoral researcher, though it might not have been clear to everyone that he was undertaking research at any particular time or even necessarily that the research directly involved them. It *was* covert in the sense that he adopted illicit means used by urban explorers to gain access to sites, and sometimes that involved misrepresenting himself both as an explorer and a researcher. Indeed, Garrett's own work suggests that, on occasion, he took the lead in the place hacking—which challenges the conventional role of the ethnographer.

11.4   Engaging in Criminal Activity as Researchers

It may be tempting to assert that researchers have a responsibility to act as law-abiding citizens. However, some legal provisions such as those associated with committing, assisting in or encouraging the commission of criminal damage in the United Kingdom have been held to cover a very wide range of behaviours (Elliott and Fleetwood 2017). There is an argument that researchers may need to engage in some illegal activities in order to gain access to and be able to undertake research in those parts of societies where breaking the law is the norm. Indeed, there is a long and celebrated history of important research within the sociology of deviance and criminology involving researchers engaging in illicit activities as part of their studies of matters such as youth gangs, drug use, and homosexuality through the Twentieth Century. More recently, researchers undertaking covert research on football hooliganism or the night-time economy (Pearson 2009; Winlow et al. 2001) have argued that breaking the law enables them to blend into the field and gain the trust of participants. In his work on criminal activity in the East End of London, British criminologist, Dick Hobbs reasoned that he had to demonstrate a '…willingness to abide by the ethics of the researched culture and not the normative ethical constraints of sociological research' and that 'a failure to adhere to these norms would have closed the research field' (1996, 7). Even within the confines of administrative criminology, such research may be important if, for example, it leads to a better understanding of and better responses by justice institutions to particular groups that could not be studied in any other way.

Like Hobbs, Pearson argued that it was necessary for covert researchers 'to act in line with research subject norms over the entire period of research if s/he wishes to retain trust and access' (2009, 248). He described how during three years of covert participant observation of football hooliganism he

> committed 'minor' offences (which I tentatively defined as those which would not cause direct physical harm to a research subject) on a weekly basis as part of the research routine. My strategy was to commit only the offences which the majority of the research subjects were committing and that I considered necessary to carry out the research. Furthermore, whilst I would commit lesser offences with regularity I would, if possible, avoid more serious ones. (Pearson 2009, 246–7)

So, in contravention of the Public Order Act, Pearson charged across a football pitch with 400 other fans following the final whistle of a match, chasing the opposing supporters and retreating when ordered back by the police. He smuggled alcohol for football supporters onto trains that had been designated as alcohol-free, and threatened a rival group in a public house (calculating that the situation would not escalate).

At some points, Garrett has argued that his group had not done anything criminal.[1] However, Garrett himself noted that 'Ethnographic research in sociology, anthropology, criminology and geography relies on the ability of the researcher to embed themselves within a community and build relations of trust within it' (quoted in Matthews 2014) and wrote that it would be impossible not to engage in trespass if researching urban explorers, as 'passive "observers" are swiftly identified, censured and disregarded in this community' (Garrett 2014b). As a result, 'My methodology then, built to satisfy both myself and my project participants, was based around doing urban exploration with them rather than speculating on it from a safe distance' (Garrett 2014a).

On the other hand, critics of such research have responded that researchers who commit crimes and risk arrest and prosecution might bring their academic disciplines, research institutions and funders into disrepute, thereby undermining the credibility of scientific research more generally among politicians, policy-makers and the general public.

However, in a later piece (Dekeyser and Garrett 2018), Garrett goes beyond the traditional instrumental argument for law-breaking to align himself with those researchers who have argued that challenging unjust laws is not just defensible but imperative. Of course, some social scientists have gone to prison rather than breach

---

[1] Festival of Dangerous Ideas, Sydney, Australia, August 2014 https://www.bradleygarrett.com/fes tival-of-dangerous-ideas/.

the confidentiality of their participants (Israel 2015). Other researchers have demonstrated against unjust laws, and most critical criminologists would not find it hard to list a range of laws that they believed we would be better off without. However, critical criminologists have not necessarily asserted their right as researchers to break the law without facing the same consequences as other citizens. The researcher as transgressor, organising pre-meditated breach of specific laws as a (not always political) expression of living life on the edge, is less common.

A more coherent argument in favour of law breaking by researchers has been made by Ferrell (2012). Ferrell has been arrested as part of a graffiti crew, convicted and sentenced to one year's probation for destruction of private property in the form of 'graffiti-vandalism' (Ferrell 1997), and arrested and tried for obstruction as part of mass action by cyclists to challenge the dominance of city streets by cars. Ferrell argued that if researchers were to understand the meaning of social activity, they could not simply observe or document; they also needed to attempt to 'understand the meaning of these interactions for those who engage in them, to participate in the emotions that animate them, and so to capture the human feel and texture of the situations they study' (1997, 223). In his statement for the defence in Garrett's case, Ferrell (2014) argued:

> if we reject this approach, we are in effect rejecting the importance of understanding the life worlds and activities of any group that may be engaged in illegal activities, or that the authorities may argue is engaged in such activities. To do so would undermine the disciplinary mandates of sociology, criminology, anthropology, and related fields, and would leave scholars, the general public, and public policy makers ignorant of a wide swath of social life.

Ferrell knowingly and intentionally took part in collective activities that broke laws, albeit often the specific laws whose nature and impact he was keen to understand. However, Ferrell's depiction of painting a piece as part of a graffiti crew, for example, differs in scale from Garrett's portrayal of himself as the planner of a wave of trespasses. In addition, the activities in which Ferrell engaged do not appear to have placed others in physical danger, and Ferrell acknowledged that the ethics of autoethnography involving violent offending might require more thought.

These arguments about the ability of people to deploy their role as researchers to defend themselves against criminal charges might become even more important in societies where on the one hand authoritarian populism mobilises support around attacks on science and research and, on the other, researchers are drawn to investigate both authoritarian politics and the use of the criminal justice system to delegitimate opposition.

As an aside, my questions about the interventionist position that researchers take as researchers, also extend to those who justify harming others while engaging in covert research on law enforcement officers. As a PhD student, Miller posed as a 'confidential informant' to narcotics officers in the United States, participating in 28 narcotics cases and setting up 'reverse sting' operations. This involved persuading people to buy illegal drugs from undercover officers. Agents would later move in to arrest the buyers and seize any of the buyer's assets or cash involved in the deal. Miller was highly critical of these operations and justified his use of covert techniques as a way of exposing 'this expensive and dysfunctional drug enforcement strategy' (Miller and Selva 1994, 323). Miller did not discuss the direct impact his work could have on suspects. Yet, Miller engaged in what other jurisdictions might term entrapment. In one case, for example, a small-time user and possible dealer of marijuana was arrested, and his cash and truck were seized. Miller and Selva acknowledged that 'the buyer might never have acted on his intentions to purchase a felonious quantity of drugs if the researcher and the agent had not presented him with such an opportunity' (1994, 324–5).

11.5 Autoethnography

As the term implies, autoethnography draws on both autobiography and ethnography. Autoethnography is a way of doing and writing research—it is both a process and a product of a systematic analysis of personal experiences in order to make sense of cultural experiences. Autoethnographies can be created by one person or collectively.

Autoethnography involves an explicit rejection of the positivist approach to science and its emphasis on objectivity and impassive neutrality, preferring to acknowledge standpoint specificity and give space to previously silenced voices, the emotional impact and therapeutic nature of research, and the researcher's impact on the research context. Autoethnography moves beyond immersion and the long-established social science practice of participant observation to document the experiences of researchers as fully engaged in the social activity. As Ferrell (2012) noted, all ethnography involves some autoethnography as many ethnographers participate in or influence the setting that they are studying, and their reflections on their own position in relation to the topic and setting help a reader assess the nature and value of their account. In ethnography, these self-reflections can be used as emotionally-evocative 'narrative hooks' to draw in the reader, before the analysis extends to matters beyond the immediate experience of the autoethnographer.

Autoethnography is not only the telling of stories, though the evocative and aesthetic way in which a story is told is important; it has to illuminate and provide new perspectives on cultural experience. For its advocates, individual and collective autoethnographies offer

> ways of producing meaningful, accessible, and evocative research grounded in personal experience, research that would sensitize readers to issues of identity politics, to experiences shrouded in silence, and to forms of representation that deepen our capacity to empathize with people who are different from us. (Ellis et al. 2011)

These positions pose significant challenges to what social scientists might traditionally have considered as being research let alone the practices of disciplines outside the social sciences. They also raise challenges for the ethics of social research.

While autoethnographies may well focus on the self, other people are often present in the narrative and just because it is the narrator's story, does not mean that the views of others carry no weight:

the rights of the 'other' in autoethnography are weighted against the interests of the self when the starting point of research is one's own sociological imagination and is likely to involve others. (Tolich 2010, 1599)

Autoethnographers often rely on retrospective consent—having encountered an experience worth recounting, they may then seek consent from other people to whom they will refer in their account. However, there is a risk that presenting a deeply personal account in which the researcher has invested considerable time and emotional labour to people with whom the autoethnographer has a strong relationship may be coercive. People may find it difficult to refuse permission to their partners, parents or children, particularly when the autoethnographer may need to publish the story for their own career advancement, a matter that their family may also be invested in.

It may be extremely difficult to disguise the identities of other people when the name of the autoethnographer is known. Even if the autoethnographer adopts a pseudonym, members of their family or close friends may well recognise others who appear in the narrative and some of the insights offered may be hurtful or damaging. Many of those whose identity might be inferred from the narrative will not have given consent—how can an autoethnographer seek consent from all those with whom he or she has come into contact and to whom he or she wishes to refer (the neighbour who plays loud music; the primary school teacher in whose class the autoethnographer was 30 years ago; the cousin who shouted random obscenities out of a car window; the mother who died)?

Critical of the failure of many autoethnographers to explore these ethical questions effectively, Tolich (2010) offered 10 foundational guidelines for ethical use of authoethnography:

1. Respect participants' autonomy and the voluntary nature of participation, and document the informed consent processes...
2. Practice 'process consent', checking at each stage to make sure participants still want to be part of the project...
3. Recognize the conflict of interest or coercive influence when seeking informed consent after writing the manuscript...
4. Consult with others...
5. Autoethnographers should not publish anything they would not show the persons mentioned in the text...
6. Beware of internal confidentiality: the relationship at risk is not with the researcher exposing confidences to outsiders, but confidences exposed among the participants or family members themselves...
7. Treat any autoethnography as an inked tattoo by anticipating the author's future vulnerability...
8. ...no story should harm others, and if harm is unavoidable, take steps to minimize harm...
9. Those unable to minimize risk to self or others should use a nom de plume...
10. Assume all people mentioned in the text will read it one day...

Over the course of his doctoral work, Garrett (2012) shifted from ethnography towards autoethnography. He 'sought to completely collapse my identity into the group, to become the researched..., to write from a life of direct experience', going

> beyond the participant/observer relationship to becoming an active producer and reproducer of the culture under study. In effect, over the course of my research I rendered myself invisible in the study group as a researcher... (2012, 44–45)

Garrett (2014a) described how while taking part in the planning of a new wave of trespass, transgressing the space of 'every under-construction skyscraper, utility, water and transportation network possible', his ability to maintain critical distance from the activity 'started to slip': 'I myself was reluctant... I also was not sure what I was doing was legal or ethical anymore in terms of my research praxis.' He also acknowledged that by 2012 he had moved towards become a 'central character' in the activities of the LCC, a position acknowledged by academic reviewers of his book:

> Urbex has attracted a huge following online, while much of the media, even those at the centre and right, have enjoyed spinning out a series of nerdy hero/playful anarchy storylines with Garrett front and centre. (Hall 2013)

It was also a matter that one urban explorer pointed out to Garrett, and that Garrett at least partly conceded in his thesis conclusion:

> I met with Marc Exp[l]o as I was rewriting the conclusion to this thesis. I told him that, as I wrote earlier, I felt I was quite lucky that I met "Team B" when I did and that I was able to integrate myself into the culture as I had done. He responded, "Brad, you didn't integrate yourself into the culture, you created the culture so that you would have something to study" (Marc Explo, January 2012). Marc's comments haunted me for weeks. Although I think most of what happened would have happened with or without me (as evidenced by what I missed over the summer of 2011 while I was away writing), there is no doubt it would have happened in a different way. Perhaps if I had not started this research, there would be no LCC. Whatever my involvement triggered, I do believe it's a vital component of my ethnographic work to acknowledge that role in the rise and fall of the "Team B" and the LCC... (Garrett 2012, 329).

In a later article, Garrett and a colleague described scaling the walls of the decommissioned Maze prison in Northern Ireland, 'sweating, bleeding hands sliding down wet, springing rope, the barking getting louder and closer' (Kindynis and Garrett 2015, 15). Only later did they reconsider the event as fit for autoethnography: 'That exploring the Maze might comprise autoethnographic "data" for a criminological journal article was, to be frank, an afterthought' (2015, 11).

11.6 Romanticisation

Beyond academic journal articles, Garrett created and co-created a series of videos about his crew's activities as a place hacker. Sometimes, this was part of his visual ethnography, sometimes part of the collective activities that some participants engaged in, sometimes possibly a benefit he was able to offer other urban explorers in exchange for his participation in the group. However, filming is also part of the performance of trespass, making public the success of his group in breaching security at iconic London sites.

A criticism made of Garrett's work is that at times it appears to become less about the nature of transgressing space and more a breathless autoethnographic exploration of adventure-seeking (Iphofen 2014). One of the more vivid examples of this in an academic journal can be found when Garrett (2012) described how as one of 'three international hobo ninjas', he 'prepared to sneak into the underworld' in Paris:

> voilà, we crossed the liminal zone of the 'known' city into a realm of illicit encounter, raw experience, playful exuberance and corporal terror. (2011, 272)

There have been several critiques of the romantic portrayal of urban exploration that can be found in the academic literature. A co-author of Garrett, Kindynis (2017: 993) argues that urban exploring has always appealed to those attracted by 'thrill-seeking, sensation-gathering, cultivating an edgy "transgressive" persona'. Kindynis is also critical of 'romantic theoretical flights of fancy' (2017: 989) exhibited among cultural social scientists who are keen to interpret new cultural forms such as urban exploration as exemplars of resistance. Indeed, Mott and Roberts (2014) note that far from being transgressive, urban exploration appears to be a celebration of able-bodied, heteronormative and white masculinity.

11.7   Balancing Harms and Benefits

While the medical ethics prescription 'do no harm' is often mentioned in discussions of research ethics, most research ethics guidelines recognise the prevalence, magnitude and distribution of harm should not be considered in isolation but as part of a consideration that encompasses both harm and benefit: 'It is commonly said that benefits and risks must be "balanced" and shown to be "in a favourable ratio"' (National Commission for the Protection of Human Subjects of Biomedical and Behavioral Research 1979).

In addition, research undertaken in the social sciences may quite legitimately and deliberately work to the detriment of research participants by revealing and critiquing their role in causing 'fundamental economic, political or cultural disadvantage or exploitation' (Economic and Social Research Council in its now superseded 2010 Framework). Similarly, researchers uncovering corruption, violence or pollution need not work to minimize harm to the corporate or institutional entities responsible for the damage though they might be expected to minimize any personal harm. At one point, Finnish guidelines also acknowledged the issue by recognizing that 'research concerning the use of power and the functioning of social institutions must not be restricted on the grounds that results can have negative effects for subjects' (National Advisory Board on Research Ethics 2009, s2.2).

Not only do risks of harms need to be commensurate with potential benefits, but sometimes researchers need to choose between competing benefits and competing harms, knowing that they only have the resources or skills to achieve some benefits and minimise some harms (Josselson 2007). These choices do not have random effects—they may both be patterned across space and demographics. In short, the choices that are made about who might benefit and how, and who might be harmed and how are also questions of distributive justice.

There are good reasons to study urban exploration and criminal trespass. Like other academics who have researched the phenomenon, Garrett interpreted trespass as a democratic, albeit not always self-aware, response to the privatisation and social control of space. One geographer, reviewing Garrett's 2013 book, wrote of the importance of documenting 'grassroots responses to a sense of stultifying cultural foreclosure, as we are funnelled through a cynically choreographed urban landscape of spectacle and consumerism' (Gandy 2015). The justification of harm in the research ethics literature is generally articulated in relation to a particular individual, group, organisation or institution rather than late-capitalism and social control in general.

The slow decay of heritage sites has been documented longitudinally by urban explorers when there appears to be little interest among or capacity within other organisations. Indeed, Garrett (2012) noted that one collection in London had caught the interest of the British Museum. As part of his work, Garrett contributed to this visual ethnography with both still photography and video images.

Criminalisation and commodification have become linked through urban exploration as the coolness associated with transgression has been deployed by companies such as Nike to promote cutting-edge attire. Surprisingly, and perhaps ironically, some other tangible benefits for the capitalist economy may flow from urban exploration. By revealing gaps in security, place-hackers have helped organisations tighten control over entry to and surveillance of sites. As with computer hackers, this seems an unlikely aim of exponents. Garrett told a journalist (Craddock 2012) and a Sydney audience that his crew would have probably been happy to advise Transport for London of the potential for security breaches if they had been asked rather than prosecuted.[2] On the other hand, Kindynis (2017) portrayed a tightening of security as an (again) ironic consequence of attempts to subvert spatial controls.

In the same Sydney speech in 2014, Garrett also suggested that media coverage of urban explorers had encouraged others to reclaim forgotten and unused spaces for public or entrepreneurial activity by stimulating tourism and other activities involving these heritage sites. Garrett said that his group had also unsuccessfully sought to encourage homeless people to access unused space for squatting.

Risk assessment is not as exciting as risk-taking and so, to compete in the media, there is a danger that more sober assessments of the risks posed to others by recreational trespass are 'sexed up'. Both Garrett and Kindynis have pointed to a one-page unclassified document purportedly published by the National Counterterrorism

---

[2] Festival of Dangerous Ideas, Sydney, Australia, August 2014 https://www.bradleygarrett.com/festival-of-dangerous-ideas/.

Center (2012) in the United States and reproduced on the Public Intelligence website.[3] This document claims that images and videos posted online by urban explorers 'could be used by terrorists to remotely identify and surveil potential targets. Advanced navigation and mapping technologies, including three-dimensional modelling and geotagging, could aid terrorists in pinpointing locations in dense urban environments'. The document was subjected to considerable derision on the internet. However, there is no reference to the document (or to urban explorers) on the website of the Office of the Director of National Intelligence where the NCTC is housed.

Unfortunately, the risks of harm to non-trespassers are not clearly addressed by Garrett in his publications—though they may well have been in any application for research ethics review—other than to point out the ridiculousness of some of the wilder claims.

However, there are more sober claims of harm caused by these activities, including those with which Garrett's group may have been involved. For example, the Vice Chairman of Friends of West Norwood Cemetery wrote that infiltration of privatised space extended to desecration of a tomb that represented a threat to public health:

> The gang also broke into the catacombs at West Norwood Cemetery, and opened up a sealed coffin. I am the person that monitors the structure of the crypt, thus they potentially exposed me to smallpox, TB and anthrax, diseases which could have still been viable in the corpse they desecrated. (Fenn 2015)

Fenn noted that the cemetery had suffered subsequently from copycat incursions.

Other agencies have maintained that by highlighting vulnerability, urban explorers have put key infrastructure at risk. John Strutton (2013), Community Safety and Crime Prevention Manager at Transport for London, argued urban explorers were causing problems for London's transport system. The organisation owed a duty of care to anyone on its properties, and even if urban explorers were unhurt there was a possibility that staff might be injured or children put at risk if access points were left open by explorers. At one point, a counter-terrorism alert had been issued when a member of the London Consolidation Crew emerged from a drain along the Olympic torch-bearing route. More troubling, train schedules would be disrupted if the organisation suspected that people were or had been inside the network overnight. In short, the risk of delaying people's travel to work distributed a multi-million-pound cost across the London economy. Strutton also criticised the sharing of information on closed internet discussion groups of how to evade security measures, as this might help other groups with more overtly disruptive agendas.

11.8 Conclusion

Part of the difficulty in critiquing Garrett's work is that it is not always clear on what basis it might be judged. As an academic study, what methodology does it

---

[3] *Urban Exploration offers insight into Critical Infrastructure Vulnerabilities*, 19 November 2012. https://info.publicintelligence.net/NCTC-UrbanExploration.pdf. Accessed 7 January 2022.

adopt—is it an ethnography or an autoethnography? It may make methodological sense to blend the two, but there are ethical consequences and, as Tolich has suggested, autoethnography is still developing responses to the ethical challenges it faces. Ground-breaking, innovative work is necessarily transgressive and contests boundaries, but code-switching between different communities of practice can be both a challenge to conventional wisdom and a way of evading accountability.

In addition, Garrett adopts various professional and personal roles—sometimes he is an ethnographer, sometimes an urban explorer, sometimes a political activist, film-maker or gonzo journalist. Analysts working in the field of research ethics are interested in his activities as an ethnographer but would not wish to use the bureaucratic processes of research ethics review to curtail his rights as a citizen to engage in political activism.

Of course, we all maintain multiple roles; no-one is 'just a researcher'. Ethnographers and autoethnographers draw on knowledge or skills gained during another role to inform their research activity. A problem for research ethicists occurs when access to data gained in one role is then used in another, particularly when access to that data would not otherwise have been afforded to a researcher. Biomedical ethics has long been concerned to separate the doctor as physician from the doctor as researcher role. In the social sciences, too, there is a danger that deliberately blurring the delineation between researcher and non-researcher roles might be considered deceptive and possibly harmful to participants as well as threatening the work of other researchers whose access may be curtailed or safety compromised (Iphofen 2013).

Acknowledgements This study draws on Israel and Gelsthorpe (2017). I am grateful to both Jeff Ferrell and Helen Kara for sharing their respective submissions to defence and prosecution counsel with me and to Ron Iphofen, Helen Kara and Robert Dingwall for their comments on earlier drafts.

References

Becker, Howard S. 2017. *Evidence*. Chicago: University of Chicago Press.
Booth, Robert. 2014. Oxford University academic who scaled shard is spared jail sentence. *The Guardian*, 23 May. https://www.theguardian.com/education/2014/may/22/oxford-university-aca demic-shard-jail-place-hacker-garrett. Accessed 2 Sep 2021.
Craddock, Adrian. 2012. Underground ghost station explorers spook the security services. *The Guardian*, 24 Feb. https://www.theguardian.com/uk/2012/feb/24/london-underground-exp lorers-security-services. Accessed 2 Sep 2021.
Dekeyser, Thomas, and Bradley L. Garrett. 2018. Ethics ≠ Law. *Area* 50: 410–417. https://doi.org/ 10.1111/area.12411.
Dingwall, Robert. 1980. Ethics and ethnography. *Sociological Review* 28 (4): 871–891.
Economic and Social Research Council, United Kingdom. 2010, revised 2012. *Framework for research ethics*. Swindon: Economic and Social Research Council. http://www.esrc.ac.uk/about-esrc/information/research-ethics.aspx. Accessed 23 Dec 2013.

Economic and Social Research Council, United Kingdom. 2015. *Framework for research ethics.* Swindon: Economic and Social Research Council. http://www.esrc.ac.uk/funding/guidance-for-applicants/research-ethics/.

Ellis, Carolyn, Tony E. Adams and Arthur P. Bochner. 2011. Autoethnography: An overview. *Forum Qualitative Sozialforschung/Forum: Qualitative Social Research* 12(1) Article 10. http://www.qualitative-research.net/index.php/fqs/article/view/1589/3095.

Elliott, Tracey, and Jennifer Fleetwood. 2017. Law for ethnographers. *Methodological Innovations* 10 (1): 1–13.

European Commission. 2010. *Guidance Note for Researchers and Evaluators of Social Sciences and Humanities Research.* http://ec.europa.eu/research/participants/data/ref/fp7/89867/social-sci ences-humanities_en.pdf. Accessed 21 Feb 2019.

Fenn, Colin. 2015. Personal correspondence with Ron Iphofen. 4th Nov.

Ferrell, Jeff. 1997. Criminological verstehen: Inside the immediacy of crime. *Justice Quarterly* 14 (1): 3–23.

Ferrell, Jeff. 2012. Research ethics in criminology. In *Sage handbook of criminological research methods,* ed. David Gadd, Susanne Karstedt, and Steven F. Messner, 218–230. London: Sage.

Ferrell, Jeff. 2014. *Statement of Witness.* 23rd April.

Ferrell, Jeff, Keith Hayward, and Jock Young. 2015. *Cultural criminology: An invitation,* 2nd ed. London: Sage.

Fountain, Jane. 1993. Dealing with data. In *Interpreting the field: Accounts of ethnography,* ed. Dick Hobbs and Tim May, 145–173. Oxford: Clarendon Press.

Gandy, Matthew. 2015. Bradley L. Garrett: Explore everything: Place-hacking the city. *International Journal of Urban and Regional Research* 39(5): 1062–1063. https://doi.org/10.1111/1468-2427. 12269.

Garrett, Bradley L. 2011. Cracking the Paris Carrières: Corporal Terror and illicit encounter under the city of light. *ACME: An International E-Journal for Critical Geographies* 10(2): 269–277.

Garrett, Bradley L. 2012. *Place hacking: Tales of urban exploration,* unpublished PhD thesis, Department of Geography, Royal Holloway, University of London. http://pure.royalholloway.ac. uk/portal/files/16913666/Place_Hacking_Bradley_L._Garrett.pdf. Accessed 9 Sep 2018.

Garrett, Bradley. 2013. *Explore everything: Place-hacking the city.* London: Verso.

Garrett, Bradley. 2014a. Undertaking recreational trespass: Urban exploration and infiltration. *Transactions of the Institute of British Geographers* 39: 1–13. https://doi.org/10.1111/tran.12001.

Garrett, Bradley. 2014b. Place-hacker Bradley Garrett: research at the edge of the law. *Times Higher Education,* 5 Jun. http://www.timeshighereducation.co.uk/story.aspx?storyCode=201 3717. Accessed 9 Jun 2014.

Hall, Tim. 2013. Explore everything: Place-hacking the city. *Times Higher Education* 28 Nov: 50.

Hobbs, Dick. 1996. *Doing the business: Entrepreneurship, detectives and the working class in the east end of London.* Oxford: Clarendon.

Iphofen, Ron. 2013. *Research ethics in ethnography/anthropology.* Brussels: European Commis-sion, DG Research and Innovation. http://ec.europa.eu/research/participants/data/ref/h2020/ other/hi/ethics-guide-ethnog-anthrop_en.pdf. Accessed 2 Sep 2021.

Iphofen, Ron. 2014. Risk management. *Times Higher Education* 3 July: 26.

Israel, Mark. 2015. *Research ethics and integrity for social scientists: Beyond regulatory compliance.* London: Sage.

Israel, Mark, and Loraine Gelsthorpe. 2017. Ethics in criminological research: A powerful force or a force for the powerful? In *Research ethics in criminology and criminal justice: Politics, dilemmas, issues and solutions,* ed. Malcolm Cowburn, Loraine Gelsthorpe, and Azrini Wahidin, 185–203. London: Routledge.

Josselson, Ruthellen. 2007. The ethical attitude in narrative research: Principles and practicalities. In *Handbook of narrative inquiry: Mapping a methodology,* ed. D. Jean Clandinin, 537–566. Thousand Oaks, CA: Sage.

Kindynis, Theo. 2017. Urban exploration: From subterranea to spectacle. *British Journal of Criminology* 57: 982–1001.

Kindynis, Theo, and Bradley L. Garrett. 2015. Entering the Maze: Space, time and exclusion in an abandoned Northern Ireland prison. *Crime Media Culture* 11 (1): 5–20.

Matthews, David. 2014. 'Place-hacker' prosecution 'attack on intellectual freedom'. *Times Higher Education*, 22 May.

Miller, J. Mitchell., and Lance H. Selva. 1994. Drug enforcement's double-edged sword: An assessment of asset forfeiture programs. *Justice Quarterly* 11 (2): 313–335.

Mott, Carrie, and Susan M. Roberts. 2014. Not Everyone Has (the) Balls: Urban exploration and the persistence of masculinist geography. *Antipode* 46: 229–245.

National Advisory Board on Research Ethics, Finland. 2009. *Ethical principles of research in the humanities and social and behavioural sciences and proposals for ethical review*. Helsinki: National Advisory Board on Research Ethics. http://www.tenk.fi/en/ethical-review-in-human-sci ences. Accessed 9 Sep 2018.

National Commission for the Protection of Human Subjects of Biomedical and Behavioral Research (NCPHSBBR). 1979. *Belmont report: Ethical principles and guidelines for the protection of human subjects of research*. Report, Department of Health, Education and Welfare, Office of the Secretary, Protection of Human Subjects, Michigan. http://www.hhs.gov/ohrp/humansubjects/ guidance/belmont.html. Accessed 28 Jan 2014.

Pearson, Geoff. 2009. The researcher as hooligan: Where 'participant' observation means breaking the law. *International Journal of Social Research Methodology* 12 (3): 243–255.

Strutton, John. 2013. Urban exploration: An emerging for challenge for 'CPTED M'?, Socially Responsive Design, 26 July. https://vimeo.com/71098376. Accessed 31 Aug 2021.

Tolich, Martin. 2010. A critique of current practice: Ten foundational guidelines for autoethnographers. *Qualitative Health Research* 20(12): 1599–1610.

Winlow, Simon, Dick Hobbs, Stuart Lister, and Philip Hadfield. 2001. Get ready to duck. Bouncers and the realities of ethnographic research on violent groups. *British Journal of Criminology* 41: 536–548.

Chapter 12
'One Health' Research Ethics in Emergency, Disaster and Zoonotic Disease Outbreaks: A Case Study from Ethiopia

Joseph M. Nguta, Kuastros M. Belaynehe, Andréia G. Arruda, Getnet Yimer, and Dónal O'Mathúna

Abstract *'One Health'* is the concept that human health and well-being are linked to the health of animals and the environment. The goals of One Health include addressing potential or existing global and transnational health risks, which require policies that are systematic, coordinated, collaborative, multidisciplinary and cross-sectoral. One Health is particularly well-suited for zoonotic diseases and emerging and re-emerging infectious diseases (EIDs). Epidemics, emergencies and disasters raise many ethical issues for all involved, including communities, responders, public health specialists and policymakers. Our case study describes ethical dilemmas encountered during an animal disease outbreak investigation in the Somali region of Ethiopia during the 2019 Coronavirus Disease (COVID-19) pandemic with concurrent drought and human conflicts. Outbreak investigations were conducted through systematic collection, analysis and evaluation of pertinent data, and results disseminated to relevant stakeholders. Our observations highlighted the importance

---

Joseph M. Nguta and Kuastros M. Belaynehe—These authors contributed equally to this work and both should be regarded as first authors

---

J. M. Nguta
Department of Public Health, Pharmacology and Toxicology, University of Nairobi, Nairobi, Kenya

K. M. Belaynehe
Epidemiology Unit, Animal Health Institute, Sebeta, Ethiopia

Emergency Centre for Transboundary Animal Diseases, Food and Agriculture Organization of the United Nations, Addis Ababa, Ethiopia

A. G. Arruda
Department of Veterinary Preventive Medicine, College of Veterinary Medicine, The Ohio State University, Columbus, OH, USA

G. Yimer
The Ohio State University, Columbus, OH, USA

D. O'Mathúna (✉)
College of Nursing and Center for Bioethics, The Ohio State University, Columbus, OH, USA
e-mail: omathuna.6@osu.edu

of addressing community humanitarian needs and potential risks to responders, including researchers, when responding to animal disease outbreaks without compromising ethical principles. Community engagement was crucial in resolving technical and ethical issues. Policy gaps related to ethical issues during animal health emergencies were observed. Our case study supports the formulation of guidelines and policies for One Health research ethics in Africa and elsewhere to strengthen capacity and ethical decision-making.

Keywords COVID-19 · One Health · Zoonosis · Outbreak investigation · Ethical dilemmas · One Health research ethics · Humanitarian issues

Acronyms

AMR	Antimicrobial resistance
CDC	Centers for Disease Control and Prevention
CIOMS	Council for International Organizations of Medical Sciences
EID	Emerging and reemerging infectious disease
MoA	Ministry of Agriculture
NAHDIC*	National Animal Health Diagnostic and Investigation Center, Ethiopia
	*NAHDIC has now changed to the Animal Health Institute (AHI)
REC	Research ethics committee
SOPs	Standard operating procedures
WHO	World Health Organization

12.1 Introduction

Infectious diseases continue to negatively impact human health and well-being, even before COVID-19 took center stage. In a sub-Saharan country such as Kenya, which has a population of 47.6 million (KNBS 2019), the top three causes of death are infectious diseases; in Ethiopia, with over 110 million people, three of the top five causes of death are infectious diseases (IHME 2019). In the past, public health responses and policies often focused on the human dimensions of infectious diseases and how they could be mitigated. In recent years, a broader approach known as '*One Health*' has received greater attention.

One Health is a multidisciplinary approach to "achieving optimal health outcomes recognizing the interconnection between people, animals, plants, and their shared environment" (CDC 2021). COVID-19 has dramatically demonstrated the global significance of emerging and reemerging infectious diseases (EIDs) and their implications for public health. One Health approaches to public health are well suited to EIDs, particularly zoonotic diseases, for both those nationally prioritized (Salyer et al. 2017) and neglected tropical diseases (Elelu et al. 2019).

Zoonotic diseases are caused by infectious agents that are present in animals and are also capable of infecting humans, with the potential of causing human illness. At least 60% of today's EIDs are of zoonotic origin, involving domestic and wild animals (Otte and Pica-Ciamarra 2021). Examples include Ebola, rabies, *Salmonella* infections, and emerging coronavirus infections. Other health risks suited to a One Health approach include those related to EIDs (Muzemil et al. 2018), for example mineral poisoning (WHO 2015; CDC 2016), food safety, antimicrobial resistance (AMR), vector-borne infectious diseases, toxicosis and pesticides (Kimani et al. 2019).

Public health initiatives taking a One Health approach have recently increased significantly. One Health has been adopted by the Centers for Disease Control and Prevention (CDC), the World Health Organization (WHO), the United Nation's Food and Agriculture Organization, and the World Organization for Animal Health (O'Mathúna et al. 2020), and the United Nations Environment Programme as of 2022. The approach is particularly well-suited for resource-limited regions of the world where people live in close proximity to animals and natural habitats. In 2018, about 100 One Health networks existed globally (Khan et al. 2018). By 2020, there were 101 One Health initiatives in East Africa alone (Fasina and Fasanmi 2020), an area regarded as one of the world's hotspots for EIDs of zoonotic origins (Kemunto et al. 2018). One Health works very well in sub-Saharan Africa as it can facilitate cross-sectoral, cross-disciplinary engagement and lead to better outcomes more economically (Fasina et al. 2020).

Regardless of where an infectious disease originates, it can quickly spread globally as demonstrated by COVID-19. Disease outbreaks continue to have devastating effects medically, economically and socially at local, regional and global levels. The West Africa Ebola outbreak of 2014–2016 cost an estimated US$2.8 billion in gross domestic product and resulted in 11,000 deaths, 80% of which could have been averted if appropriate funding and response had been available two months earlier (GPMB 2019). Factors such as climate change, increased ease and speed of cross-border movements, emergence of new pathogens, and re-emergence of endemic pathogens pose increased risks to global health security. Many types of events, including epidemics and pandemics, climate change and natural disasters, industrial accidents and armed conflict, can create emergencies that impact the health of ecosystems, animals and humans. All of these point to the global significance of One Health research, practice and policy, and the importance of coordinated standard operating procedures (SOPs) to address EIDs. Developing such policies is challenging given the variety of disciplines that need to inform these areas.

12.2   One Health Ethics

Public health practice and research, particularly within veterinary medicine, has increasingly adopted One Health approaches. As with any area of public health practice or research, applying One Health approaches may lead to ethical dilemmas and challenges, but they have received little attention from bioethics (Johnson and Degeling 2019). This has been identified as a hindrance to the implementation of One Health policies in East Africa (Destoumieux-Garzón et al. 2018). Even in a country like the Netherlands, known for the strength of its bioethics research into emerging areas of research, the systems for tracking and responding to EIDs were found to be "not well equipped to handle moral dilemmas" and their One Health professionals to "have little ethical knowledge" (van Herten et al. 2020). Because One Health projects involve human, animal and environmental dimensions, different policies from different agencies are commonly applicable, and ethics and regulatory approvals may be required from several committees, sometimes in different countries (Ladbury et al. 2017). Part of the challenge here arises from the very nature of the One Health interdisciplinary approach. Individual researchers and policymakers may be familiar with the ethics of human subject research, or animal research or environmental studies within their own expertise, but not across all areas or with ethics at the points of intersection. There is some irony here, as the term bioethics stems from the work of Fritz Jahr in 1927 when he coined the term *Bio-Ethik* to address ethical obligations to all living beings, humans, animals or plants (Sass 2007). Additional ethical challenges arise when One Health practice and research is initiated due to outbreaks, which require rapid emergency responses. These conditions may overlap with other emergencies and disasters, such as when an outbreak occurs in a refugee camp with people displaced due to war. All of these factors add further complexities to the ethical issues, but heighten the importance of exploring them in order to inform policymaking in this area.

Our research team formed to explore the ethical issues that arise with One Health approaches to public health practice and research. Our team includes One Health researchers and practitioners based in Kenya, Ethiopia and the USA. We have conducted research into the views of researchers, ethics committee members and regulatory bodies about ethics in One Health research in Africa. In this chapter, we present a case study collected by the team during an animal disease outbreak investigation in Ethiopia. The case study demonstrates some of ethical issues that may arise with a One Health approach to public health. From this, combined with preliminary findings from our research, we make some recommendations for One Health policymakers regarding One Health ethics.

12.3   The Case Study

This case study explores ethical dilemmas encountered during investigation into an outbreak of animal disease, hereafter referred to as 'outbreak investigation,' in the Somali region of Ethiopia. The study region at the time was challenged with a triple burden of armed human conflict, the COVID-19 pandemic, and drought due to shortage of rain, and therefore the outbreak investigation took place in the context of concurrent humanitarian crises. The outbreak occurred among pastoralist communities whose livelihoods in Ethiopia depend entirely on their livestock, including sheep, goats and camels. Pastoralists live in areas where crops are difficult to grow due to the arid environment. Some pastoralists are semi-settled and travel during certain seasons to graze their livestock and in search of water, while others are permanently settled with some family members traveling to find grazing pasture and water, while others are constantly moving. The movements can lead to groups crossing regional and/or national boundaries. The close relationship between pastoralists and their animals increases the possibility of contracting zoonotic diseases from animals, mainly through consumption of unpasteurized milk and undercooked animal products (Megersa et al. 2011; Ayim-Akonor et al. 2020). Long-standing community practices related to animals can sometimes be at odds with health promotion or research guidelines, which can lead to challenges that require careful negotiation.

During the first week of February 2021, the Ethiopian Ministry of Agriculture (MoA) Epidemiology Directorate received a disease outbreak alert of an unknown disease affecting sheep and goats, characterized by sudden mortality. A few camel deaths were also reported. This information was immediately communicated to the then national referral laboratory, the National Animal Health Diagnostic and Investigation Centre (NAHDIC), under the Ethiopian MoA. NAHDIC was asked to participate in the investigation of this unknown disease and a team with members from different sectors of the laboratory was established. A multidisciplinary team composed of epidemiologists, microbiologists, veterinarians and laboratory technicians from NAHDIC and MoA were sent to the outbreak area.

The outbreak investigation was conducted in Liben Zone, which is one of the eleven Zones of the Somali regional state of Ethiopia, as shown in Fig. 12.1. In Ethiopia, the government administration units are named, in decreasing size, Federal, Region, Zone, Woreda, and Kebele. A multi-stage sampling approach was used for the investigation by selecting two districts, Dollo Addo Woreda and Bokolmanyo Woreda. Dollo Addo Woreda sits where three countries have their borders, namely, Kenya, Somalia and Ethiopia. The other site, Bokolmanyo Woreda, hosts one of the largest refugee camps in the Somali regional state, and zoonotic animal diseases are common within the residents. Animals health experts from Dollo Addo Woreda joined the NAHDIC and MoA outbreak investigation team.

The Liben Zone is part of an area frequently affected by drought since it experiences a short rainy season. Vegetation cover is scarce for small ruminants to feed on, with the exception of small patches along the river Dawa. The outbreak investigation took place at a time when the population was facing food shortages due to prevailing

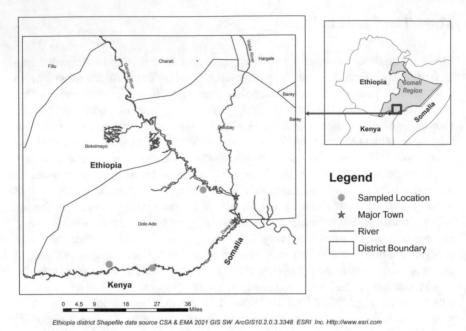

Fig. 12.1 Geospatial Imaging System (GIS) map of the animal disease outbreak investigation area, created using ArcGIS 10 software

drought and the loss of their main source of income because of the massive death of goats and sheep. In the area, practices including poor grazing management, traditional animal husbandry practices, and having livestock present within the household environment increase the potential for the occurrence of zoonotic infectious diseases. In addition, unrestricted movement of livestock across the porous borders and the presence of wild animals within the same ecosystem of farm animals are frequently noticed, again forming ideal conditions for the spread of zoonotic diseases.

The first step in the outbreak investigation was to design an implementable plan for this specific investigation. Upon arrival, the NAHDIC team conducted informational meetings with different regional officers, and zonal livestock and pastoral development officers. Interviews about the situation were conducted at many levels starting with Regional bureau heads and then with Zonal animal health focal personnel. The Zonal-level livestock health focal person arranged an interview session with two Woreda level animal health experts and three Kebele chairpersons, one person from each Kebele where the outbreak occurred. The Kebele chairperson, who knows the local pastoralists, has the responsibility to report to Woreda officials on animal health and public health-related issues and concerns happening in the Kebele. These reports are passed on to both Zonal and Region levels, finally reaching the Federal level.

After discussions with officials, engagement with the community began with local Kebele administrators and religious leaders. Each Kebele chairperson contacted the local pastoralists and arranged a meeting with the religious leader within each

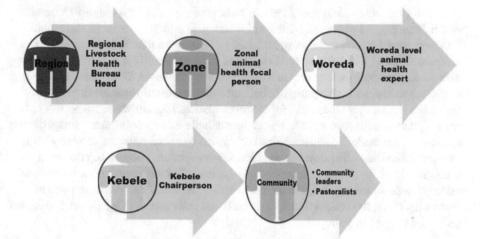

Fig. 12.2 Levels of communication during disease investigation

Kebele. The religious leaders later engaged the rest of the pastoralists and the local community was informed of the investigation's objectives and methods, and later of the investigation outcomes. The channels of communication are shown in Fig. 12.2. The community was consulted and engaged in the outbreak investigation, assisting the investigation team with collection of demographic and epidemiological data and the collection of biological samples.

In each Kebele, during sample collection, the pastoralists were interviewed to collect information about the animal disease and any abrupt climatic or environmental changes that occurred in the recent past. In some situations, the Kebele chairperson served as an interpreter during "question and answer" sessions. The engagement of the community facilitated the collection of sensitive information, such as the number of livestock per household, the number of family members in the household, how animals were used for food, how dead animals were disposed of and the numbers of pregnant animals. Communities were also engaged as they guided the investigation team on which sites to sample or not considering logistical (e.g. accessibility to roads and transportation) and security concerns.

Consent for the outbreak investigation was obtained verbally in culturally appropriate ways involving dialogue between pastoralist community leaders and the investigation team. Verbal consent was also obtained when community members assisted in handling and restraining their animals for purposes of sample collection. The observed clinical signs presented by affected animals included sudden onset of disease, diarrhea, coughing, recumbency, shivering and death. Although clinical symptomatology varied from one Kebele to another, abortion in the mid trimester was a common feature in sheep and goats. Among the twenty two Kebeles in Dollo Addo Woreda, three Kebeles reported severe disease outbreak with massive mortality in sheep and goats. In addition, a similar outbreak was reported in the Bokolmanyo Woreda, which borders Ethiopia and Kenya along river Dawa.

During the outbreak investigation in both areas, a total of 44 sheep (38 males and 6 females), 42 goats (38 males and 4 females) and 10 camels (2 males and 8 females) were examined and samples taken to investigate the cause of the unknown disease. Clinical and laboratory data would help to identify a potential zoonotic disease and samples were collected for this purpose. However, lack of resources (e.g. cold chain maintenance for sample collection and transportation) and lack of financial resources were major challenges for the investigation. In addition, retrospective data from human health care facilities were unavailable due to poor data management systems. The descriptive and interview data which were collected are currently being analyzed with the aim of developing suitable interventions and a mitigation plan for potential future outbreaks. Nevertheless, the investigation identified a number of ethical issues which we report in the next section. While this investigation was not a research project, the ethical issues identified have relevance for One Health research and point to gaps in policy.

12.4   Analysis of the Case Study

The case study notes how community engagement occurred throughout the outbreak investigation and was a key component to addressing ethical issues. Once the community understood the study objectives and its potential benefits, it became easier to navigate several processes, for example interviewing community members to obtain more information about the outbreak. Potential security risks were also minimized; the community was directly involved in identifying trusted guides, coordinating visits to different homesteads, provision of disease history, and identification of affected animals. This facilitated the disease investigation and would be important during deployment of remedial measures to address further loss of animals. The community continued to engage with investigators in designing possible interventions and a mitigation plan that would decrease further animal losses from potential future outbreaks. The plan would entail immediate reporting once disease symptoms are seen in the animals.

Our case study demonstrates the value and importance of community engagement. At the same time, such discussions take time to conduct, particularly when involving various officials, community leaders and pastoralists themselves. The time required may need to be balanced against the need to initiate investigations quickly. This engagement for outbreak investigations typically leads to informal agreements from pastoralists to participate in the investigation. However, some pastoralists did not agree to participate, possibly due to a lack of understanding of scientific approaches to disease investigation (although further work is needed to understand the reasons for non-participation). Interestingly, other pastoralists allowed blood to be drawn from some of their animals, but then stopped allowing more of their flock to be sampled for unknown reasons. Scientifically, this can compromise the thoroughness and consistency of sample collection. Yet, overruling the pastoralists' preferences would not be ethically acceptable and could have negatively impacted current or future collaboration.

Additional ethical challenges associated with working with pastoralist communities were observed during the disease investigation. The continuous movement of the pastoralists for grazing pasture and water led to difficulties involving the community, especially at the beginning, making it difficult to help all communities facing humanitarian crises.

The investigation into an animal disease outbreak claiming the lives of many animals was further complicated by concurrent crises including drought, conflict, and the COVID-19 pandemic. The potential risks to the investigators needed to be considered since the investigation was being carried out in a region characterized by ongoing conflict. After the decision was made to carry out the investigation, security for the team had to be prioritized and monitored, and became a crucial ethical consideration. Conducting investigations during armed conflict can also put local communities at risk if their engagement with the investigative team is perceived as aligning themselves with one side or another of the conflicting parties.

The outbreak investigation has led to additional ethical dilemmas now that data has been collected. Investigation results are reported to the Federal offices, which then communicate recommendations to local officials who discuss them with the community. Some investigators considered whether some of the data (epidemiological or qualitative interview reports) could be published to inform One Health research and public health practice. At the same time, some investigators could use data to contribute to work they are undertaking towards research degrees. In both situations, the lack of formal research ethics approval prior to undertaking the investigation would likely preclude such uses of this data. Outbreak investigations require an approval letter (support letter) attesting that a team of experts is being officially dispatched to the outbreak area. This can be obtained within days from the MoA and NAHDIC, but no such mechanism exists for research. However, if formal research ethics approval had been sought, it likely would have delayed the investigation for weeks or months during which time the outbreak could have had much more widespread impact. However, the type of in-depth ethical review available for research is not available for outbreak investigations. If it was, it could help ensure that best ethical practice occurs and avoid potential ethical dilemmas and concerns. Such approvals are further complicated with One Health research where animal, human and environmental ethical issues may have required approvals from a number of different committees. Further complexity and delays would have been added if the investigations required following the pastoralists into Kenya or Somalia, the countries bordering the investigation area.

12.5   Lessons Learned from the Case Study for Research Ethics

While the outbreak investigation described in this case study was not a research project, it has implications for research ethics. Many of the activities carried out during an outbreak investigation are also conducted during One Health research and therefore raise similar ethical issues. We identified some of the same ethical issues in another case study involving research in Ethiopia (Yimer et al. 2020). Community engagement was central to how that research project, and this animal outbreak investigation, addressed the ethical issues, and is increasingly advanced as an important aspect of research ethics (CIOMS 2021). We believe that community engagement is also crucial for ethics in human outbreak investigations, public health surveillance, and One Health research in general. Maintaining good relationships with the impacted community is crucial for building trust, promoting respect and ensuring that interventions and mitigation plans are more likely to be adopted and implemented.

Those involved in One Health projects need both to be culturally sensitive to important elements of other cultures and to be flexible enough to adapt to the community's culture while carrying out their investigations. These are important ethical principles that can be applied to a wide variety of One Health practices to help address ethical dilemmas and promote respect for the community (CIOMS 2021). Various strategies have been proposed to promote community engagement, including engaging trusted community members, formation of community advisory boards, and developing formal plans for sustained engagement with the community. Continuous animal movement along the porous land borders between countries also poses a risk for zoonotic and other EIDs. The cross-border situation also complicated the situation with local and regional officials involved from different countries, each with their own approach to investigations and approval systems.

Our case study also highlights one problem with existing approaches to One Health research ethics governance and policies which needs to be avoided if outbreak investigations are to be conducted efficiently. Our case study identified ways that an ethics review and approval mechanism might have helped to avoid some ethical challenges and strengthen ethics features of the investigation. However, existing research ethics procedures would likely have introduced unacceptable delays to initiating the investigation. Similar concerns have been expressed about initiating ethics approval mechanisms for research (Ladbury et al. 2017). Furthermore, the investigation involved animal, human and environmental aspects, which could require approvals from multiple committees or that various experts would need to sit on a multidisciplinary One Health ethics review committee. Additional challenges would arise if the committees were not located in the same place, making ethical approval difficult when the Liben Zone community required urgent assistance. In this particular case study, the cross-border situation added further complexity, with the possibility that ethical approvals could be needed in up to three countries. This points to the importance of SOPs, guidelines and protocols to guide ethical review of One

Health projects during emergencies like disease outbreaks, regardless of whether these are animal or human disease investigations, public health surveillance, or formal research projects. These mechanisms must include ways that reviews can be initiated at short notice and completed quickly without compromising their rigor. This requires that people reviewing such projects are thoroughly familiar with the relevant scientific, ethical and cultural issues involved. Such procedures should also involve ways that cross-border communication and consistency can be achieved, especially for emergency situations. Thus, our findings have important implications for policymakers.

12.6 Implications and Recommendations for Policymakers

One Health research ethics challenges associated with outbreak investigations in pastoral communities were observed during the disease investigation. Although all research, including outbreak investigations should abide by the foundational ethical principles established by relevant research bodies, this was difficult to do while investigating this animal disease outbreak, which generated a number of ethical dilemmas. We realized that the existing ethical guidelines were not adaptable to certain research methods, cultures, and contexts, making it challenging to design and implement studies in pastoral areas, especially at times of zoonoses, disasters, pandemics and animal health emergencies.

To achieve the goals of One Health and address potential or existing global and transnational health risks, policies should be systematic, coordinated, collaborative, multidisciplinary and cross-sectoral (Kimani et al. 2019; Yasobant et al. 2019). The process of systematically collecting, consolidating, analyzing, and evaluating pertinent data, as well as disseminating results to relevant stakeholders during zoonotic disease outbreaks, emergencies and disasters requires a One Health approach to safeguard the health of humans, animals and the environment. Whether such procedures are formally defined as research, public health surveillance or outbreak investigations is not as important as whether they occur effectively, ethically, efficiently and in a timely manner. This implies that ethical conduct of emerging disease investigations requires ethical input and oversight by those familiar with and competent in animal, human and environmental ethics. Community and cultural input is also vital.

These requirements complicate ethical issues since such projects will often involve human, animal and environmental factors that are regulated and overseen by several governmental departments. Given the cross-border nature of emerging infectious and zoonotic diseases, such as rift valley fever, brucellosis, rabies and COVID-19, approvals may be needed from a number of countries. Outbreak investigations such as the one described in this case study would also require ethical approval within a short period of time to limit the potential harm to animals, humans and the environment, and inform potential interventions and mitigation plans as soon as possible. The Ebola outbreak and the COVID-19 pandemic have highlighted the importance of initiating relevant research quickly and at the same time ensuring that ethical review remains rigorous and thorough (O'Mathúna et al. 2020). Guidelines are needed for when One Health projects would require full review or exemption from review, or some form of pre-review, especially during zoonotic disease outbreaks, emergencies, and disasters. All of these factors require careful consideration by policymakers to ensure that whatever policies and procedures are developed will address each element of these complex scenarios. One of the problems with existing research ethics policies is that most have been designed for non-emergency situations and well-resourced settings (Destoumieux-Garzón et al. 2018).

We also recommend the development of policies and support programs that would:

- enhance the ethical decision-making skills of One Health investigators and researchers, reviewers and regulators;
- strengthen the capacity of One Health practitioners, researchers, reviewers and regulators through training in One Health ethics through various programs ranging from short courses to full degree programs;
- support the formulation of guidelines, policies and SOPs to guide ethical review of One Health projects (of various types) during disease outbreaks, emergencies and pandemics, especially zoonotic ones;
- allow communities to engage in projects from inception, during execution and into final dissemination of results and designing intervention plans;
- lead to the creation of ethical review committees with multidisciplinary expertise to assure critical review of projects at the interface of human, animal and environmental health; and
- promote training of One Health reviewers on ethical issues specific to One Health.

Community engagement and cultural sensitivity must be included as essential elements of One Health practice and research. This should be especially prominent in any ethics-related policies for One Health. Guidelines should include recommendations for practical ways to promote community engagement and develop cultural sensitivity, and data should be collected on the effectiveness and acceptability of various approaches. Community engagement should also be encouraged as a way of resolving ethical dilemmas or concerns that arise during One Health investigations, particularly during disease outbreaks, disasters, and other emergencies when ethical approvals are granted more rapidly than normal. Ethics policies that promote community engagement should be seen as an important way to inform communities about the importance of One Health to their health and empower communities to ensure that their needs and concerns are addressed through outbreak investigations, public health surveillance and research.

Acknowledgements The authors are grateful to the National Institutes of Health Fogarty International Center (NIH-FIC) for supporting the current study (Award Number: 3D43TW008650-08S1). We also thank the European Union Health of Ethiopian Animals for Rural Development (HEARD) project and National Animal Health Diagnostic and Investigation Center (NAHDIC) for the financial support to conduct the animal disease outbreak investigation.

Conflict of Interest The authors declare that the case study was conducted in the absence of any commercial or financial relationships that could be construed as a potential conflict of interest.

References

Ayim-Akonor, Matilda, Ralf Krumkamp, Jürgen May, and Eva Mertens. 2020. Understanding attitude, practices and knowledge of zoonotic infectious disease risks among poultry farmers in Ghana. *Veterinary Medicine and Science* 6 (3): 631–638. https://doi.org/10.1002/vms3.257.

CDC. 2016. Lead poisoning investigation in northern Nigeria. https://www.cdc.gov/onehealth/in-action/lead-poisoning.html. Accessed 16 Oct 2021.

CDC. 2021. One Health. https://www.cdc.gov/onehealth/index.html. Accessed 16 Oct 2021.

CIOMS. 2021. Clinical research in resource-limited settings. https://cioms.ch/publications/product/clinical-research-in-low-resource-settings. Accessed 16 Oct 2021.

Destoumieux-Garzón, Delphine, Patrick Mavingui, Gilles Boetsch, Jérôme Boissier, Frédéric Darriet, Priscilla Duboz, et al. 2018. The One Health concept: 10 years old and a long road ahead. *Frontiers in Veterinary Science* 5: 14. https://doi.org/10.3389/fvets.2018.00014.

Elelu, Nusirat, Julius O. Aiyedun, Ibraheem G. Mohammed, Oladapo O. Oludairo, Ismail A. Odetokun, Kaltume M. Mohammed, James O. Bale, and Saka Nuru. 2019. Neglected zoonotic diseases in Nigeria: Role of the public health veterinarian. *Pan African Medical Journal* 32: 36. https://doi.org/10.11604/pamj.2019.32.36.15659.

Fasina, F.O., and O. G. Fasanmi. 2020. The One Health landscape in sub-Saharan African countries. Nairobi, Kenya: International Livestock Research Institute. https://www.ilri.org/publicati ons/one-health-landscape-sub-saharan african-countries. Accessed 16 Oct 2021.

Fasina, Folorunso O., Niwael Mtui-Malamsha, Gladys R. Mahiti, Raphael Sallu, Moses OleNeselle, Bachana Rubegwa, et al. 2020. Where and when to vaccinate? Interdisciplinary design and evaluation of the 2018 Tanzanian anti-rabies campaign: Biogeography-based vaccination planning. *International Journal of Infectious Diseases* 95: 352–360. https://doi.org/10.1016/j.ijid.2020.03.037.

GPMB-Global Preparedness Monitoring Board. 2019. *A World at risk: Annual report on global preparedness for health emergencies.* Geneva: World Health Organization.

IHME–Institute for Health Metrics and Evaluation. 2019. Kenya. http://www.healthdata.org/kenya

Johnson, Jane, and Chris Degeling. 2019. Does One Health require a novel ethical framework? *Journal of Medical Ethics* 45: 239–243. https://doi.org/10.1136/medethics-2018-105043.

Kemunto, Naomi, Eddy Mogoa, Eric Osoro, Austin Bitek, M. Kariuki Njenga, and S. M. Thumbi. 2018. Zoonotic disease research in East Africa. *BMC Infectious Diseases* 18:545. https://doi.org/10.1186/s12879-018-3443-8

Khan, Mishal S., Peregrine Rothman-Ostrow, Julia Spencer, Nadeem Hasan, Mirzet Sabirovic, Afifah Rahman-Shepherd, et al. 2018. The growth and strategic functioning of One Health networks: A systematic analysis. *Lancet Planetary Health* 2: e264-273. https://doi.org/10.1016/S2542-5196(18)30084-6.

Kimani, T., S. Kiambi, S. Eckford, J. Njuguna, Y. Makonnen, et al. 2019. Expanding beyond zoonoses: The benefits of a national One Health coordination mechanism to address antimicrobial resistance and other shared health threats at the human-animal-environment interface in Kenya. *Revue Scientifique et Technique* 38 (1): 155–171. https://doi.org/10.20506/rst.38.1.2950.

KNBS–Kenya National Bureau of Statistics. 2019. 2019 Kenya Population and Housing Census. Volume IV: Distribution of Population by Socio-Economic Characteristics. https://www.knbs.or.ke/?wpdmpro=2019-kenya-population-and-housing-census-volume-iv-distribution-of-popula tion-by-socio-economic-characteristics. Accessed 18 Jun 2022.

Ladbury, Georgia, Kathryn J. Allan, Sarah Cleaveland, Alicia Davis, William A. de Glanville, Taya L. Forde, et al. 2017. One Health research in northern Tanzania–challenges and progress. *East African Health Research Journal* 1 (1): 8–18. https://pubmed.ncbi.nlm.nih.gov/34308154/.

Megersa, Bekele, Demelash Biffa, Fufa Abunna, Alemayehu Regassa, Jacques Godfroid, and Eystein Skjerve. 2011. Seroprevalence of brucellosis and its contribution to abortion in cattle, camel, and goat kept under pastoral management in Borana, Ethiopia. *Tropical Animal Health and Production* 43 (3): 651–656. https://doi.org/10.1007/s11250-010-9748-2.

Muzemil, Abdulazeez, Olubunmi G. Fasanmi, and Folorunso O. Fasina. 2018. African perspectives: Modern complexities of emerging, re-emerging, and endemic zoonoses. *Journal of Global Health* 8 (2): 020310. https://jogh.org/documents/issue201802/jogh-08-020310.pdf.

O'Mathúna, Dónal. P., Andréia G. Arruda, and Getnet Yimer. 2020. One Health research ethics. *Ethiopian Journal of Health Development* 34 (4): 232–234.

Otte, Joachim, and Ugo Pica-Ciamarra. 2021. Emerging infectious zoonotic diseases: The neglected role of food animals. *One Health* 13: 100323. https://doi.org/10.1016/j.onehlt.2021.100323.

Salyer, Stephanie J., Rachel Silver, Kerri Simone, and Casey B. Behravesh. 2017. Prioritizing zoonoses for global health capacity building–Themes from One Health Zoonotic Disease Workshops in 7 countries, 2014–2016. *Emerging Infectious Diseases* 23 (13): S55–S64. https://doi.org/10.3201/eid2313.170418.

Sass, Hans-Martin. 2007. Fritz Jahr's 1927 concept of bioethics. *Kennedy Institute of Ethics Journal* 17 (4): 279–295. https://doi.org/10.1353/ken.2008.0006.

van Herten, Joost, Suzanne Buikstra, Bernice Bovenkerk, and Elsbeth Stassen. 2020. Ethical decision-making in zoonotic disease control. How do One Health strategies function in the Netherlands? *Journal of Agricultural and Environmental Ethics* 33: 239–259. https://doi.org/10.1007/s10806-020-09828-x.

WHO. 2015. Lead exposure in African children: Contemporary sources and concerns. https://apps.who.int/iris/handle/10665/200168. Accessed 30 Aug 2022.

Yasobant, Sandul, Krupali Patel, and Deepak Saxena. 2019. Hastening One Health collaboration in Gujarat, India: A SWOT analysis. *Journal of Public Health Policy and Planning* 3 (2): 22–24.

Yimer, Getnet, Wondwossen Gebreyes, Arie Havelaar, Jemal Yousuf, Sarah McKune, Abdulmuen Mohammad, and Dónal O'Mathúna. 2020. Community engagement and building trust to resolve ethical challenges during humanitarian crises: Experience from the CAGED Study. *Conflict and Health* 14: 68. https://doi.org/10.1186/s13031-020-00313-w.

Chapter 13
Artificial Intelligence (AI) in a Time of Pandemics: Developing Options for the Ethical Governance of COVID-19 AI Applications

Mihalis Kritikos

Abstract This chapter analyses the various applications of artificial intelligence (AI) developed in the context of the COVID-19 pandemic and examines the range of ethical questions that their multi-level deployment may raise. Within this frame, the author sheds light on the challenges posed by the fast-tracking authorization of some of the AI systems and pays particular attention to the form and shape that 'emergency response' in the field of ethics has taken in order to cope with these extraordinary challenges and the ethical practices that have been developed thus far. The chapter will also provide a detailed set of policy suggestions to overcome these challenges with a special focus on the need to develop an emergency ethics framework that will allow policy-makers to authorize the deployment of AI-powered tools in a responsible and trustworthy manner.

Keywords Artificial intelligence · Research ethics · COVID-19 · Ethics-by-design · Privacy · Ethics review

13.1 Introduction

The impact of the COVID-19 pandemic on AI development and the possible impact of AI on solving problems created by the outbreak has been multifaceted. More than 18 months after the declaration of the COVID-19 outbreak as a pandemic, AI seems to have been changing the way disease outbreaks are tracked, mitigated and managed at different levels. Since the outbreak of this pandemic, international organisations and scientific centers have been using AI to track the epidemic in real-time, accelerate the development of drugs, and articulate an effective and targeted response. Throughout the pandemic, AI proved to be a cross-cutting tool that is used in different ways and can play an essential role in recognizing, explaining, and predicting infection patterns.

M. Kritikos (✉)
Centre for Digitalisation, Democracy and Innovation, Brussels School of Governance,
Vrije Universiteit Brussel, Brussels, Belgium
e-mail: mihail.kritikos@gmail.com

D. O'Mathúna and R. Iphofen (eds.), *Ethics, Integrity and Policymaking*, Research Ethics Forum 9, https://doi.org/10.1007/978-3-031-15746-2_13

In view of the data-driven character of the COVID-19 pandemic, the use of AI applications has been rather intensive in healthcare settings as countries seek to understand, find cures, develop vaccines and perform conventional data analysis that is at the heart of the COVID-19 response. Although most of the machine learning applications were deployed during the COVID-19 pandemic without going through any prior authorization process, their actual impact is likely to have been modest.

AI's wide-reaching scientific capacity also raises a diverse array of ethical challenges and questions that have disrupted the operation of the traditional ethical governance schemes. The ethical challenges caused by the application of AI in this particular public health emergency context relate mostly to AI-powered restrictive enforcement measures that include domestic containment strategies without due process and the processing of vast amounts of health data in the frame of fussy algorithmic decision-making procedures without informed consent. These challenges have been accentuated by the lack of data needed to train algorithms that would be reflective of the needs of local populations, take local patterns into account, and ensure equity and fairness.

13.2 Main Applications

A scan of the technological horizon in the context of COVID-19 illustrates that the number of AI-based applications has increased considerably for different aspects of outbreak response: early warning, data gathering and analysis, monitoring, movement surveillance, automating aspects of diagnosis and prognosis (Malgieri 2020), developing vaccines, and tracing of digital contacts (Bullock et al. 2020). The breadth of applications ranges from piloting of drones that delivered medical supplies to remote regions and of robots to disinfect hospitals (McCall 2020) to the creation of health equipment databases that monitored the availability of assets in national health systems (Van der Schaar et al. 2020).

More concretely, the main warnings about the novel coronavirus were raised by AI systems more than a week before official information about the epidemic was released. Since then, AI systems have been deployed to help detect and diagnose or slow the virus' spread through surveillance and contact tracing (Berditchevskaia and Peach 2020) and to improve early warning tools through the development of AI-powered passenger locator forms (Kritikos 2020a) and the monitoring of body temperature through AI-based fever detection systems (Kritikos 2020b). The use of data in algorithmic processes has also helped many countries to prioritize healthcare resources in healthcare settings.

AI has also been used to understand and predict the virus's RNA secondary structure (Tang et al. 2020) and accelerate medical research on drugs and treatments via AI's capacity to search large databases quickly and process vast amounts of medical data essentially accelerating the development of a drug and enabling a quicker and deeper analysis of the genetic sequence of SARS-CoV-2, the virus causing COVID-19. AI can also process vast amounts of unstructured text data to predict the number of potential new cases by area and which populations will be most at risk, as well as evaluate and optimise strategies for controlling the spread of the epidemic.

This expansive spectrum of AI-supported interventions demonstrates the special role that AI systems have played at different stages of the pandemic. However, by focusing on AI applications, the chapter does not aim to underline techno-solutionism or, in other words, the idea that new and emerging technologies could solve global health problems, such as the current pandemic, on their own. Instead, by examining the way AI has been used throughout the pandemic, it argues that the use of general AI has been rather intensive in various domains of the pandemic.

13.3 Ethical Challenges

The ethical challenges related to the deployment of AI solutions at unprecedented speed and scale in the context of the pandemic touch upon the protection of privacy and autonomy, possible algorithmic bias and the informational asymmetries between citizens and governments and big tech companies across Europe and the globe. Striking a balance between the need to protect public health and promote benefi- cence and at the same time safeguard individual privacy and autonomy has been an extremely difficult and complicated policy exercise in the context of the pandemic.

Matters of security and public safety can end up taking precedence over individual rights in the context of severe health crises and policy-makers need to constantly consider trade-offs between privacy and public health given the dynamic character of the disease. The terms and conditions under which AI applications such as contact tracing, thermal imaging and passenger locator forms need to be deployed illustrate the tensions and the complexity when attempting to protect multiple public interests under extreme time pressure.

At the same time, the responsible use of data has become a major ethical challenge in the COVID-19 pandemic. Use of AI, whether for medical purposes or for epidemi- ological modelling, can be extremely sensitive, with implications for the personal privacy and security of individuals and groups. The use of AI and data-intensive applications in an emergency context raises a vast range of ethical questions about the necessity, evidence, and proportionality of the respective technological interven- tion as it may lead to the temporary suspension of fundamental rights and/or a 'new normal' of eroded rights and liberties. In addition, there are concerns that data used to fight COVID-19 can be subverted for other non-medical purposes.

The massive use of AI tracking and surveillance tools in the context of this outbreak (Kim 2020), combined with the current fragmentation in the ethical gover- nance of AI, could pave the way for wider and more permanent use of these surveil- lance technologies, leading to a situation known as 'mission creep' whereby public authorities may continue collecting sensitive information well beyond the emergency.

Other ethical considerations that relate to the use of AI in the context of the current pandemic concern the needs of vulnerable populations and issues of fairness and inclusion in the training of AI-based systems. This ethical hazard is, in fact, made worse by the disproportionately harmful effects of the COVID-19 pandemic on disadvantaged and vulnerable communities and the challenges in translating AI models to reflect local healthcare environments (Luengo-Oroz et al. 2020).

Given that the efficacy of AI systems heavily depends on the reliability and relevance of the data available, collecting and processing sufficient data for accurate monitoring, decision-making, and diagnosis has been extremely challenging in the context of the current pandemic. For that purpose, sharing data between governments and international organisations has been a crucial factor for the creation of credible and trustworthy databases.

These challenges have been augmented by the relatively immature state of most AI applications, technical limitations, and the lack of supporting ICT infrastructure and interoperability, security and standardization issues. Current processes for ethics and risk assessment around uses of AI are still relatively immature, and the urgency of a crisis highlights their limitations. Prevailing gaps in digital maturity across hospitals, regions, and countries may also act as roadblocks to accessing data of sufficient quality and quantity to pick up generalizable and transportable signals from target populations. Moreover, the use of AI in sectors such as radiological imaging is relatively new, and codes of ethics and practice for use of AI in imaging are just now being contemplated by the medical community. Current processes for ethics and risk assessment encompassing uses of AI are still relatively immature, and the urgency of a crisis of this magnitude highlights their limitations.

In addition, AI models may have differential impacts and disproportionate effects across subpopulations and on society in general, with harmful consequences that are difficult to predict in advance. A further concern is that the lack of transparency in AI systems used to aid decision-making around COVID-19 may make it nearly impossible for the decisions of governments and public officials to be subject to public scrutiny and lead to blurred accountability schemes.

13.4   Policy and Legal Responses

The challenges associated with the deployment of AI solutions have exerted undue pressure on traditional legal structures and ethical governance frameworks alike given the need to strike a balance between a cautious approach and the need to deploy technological solutions at scale. Circumstances of a public health crisis such as the COVID-19 pandemic may place processes of deliberatively balancing and prioritizing conflicting or competing values under extreme pressure to yield decisions that generate difficult trade-offs between equally inviolable principles.

Indeed, the international health emergency related to the pandemic had a huge impact on the process of review and authorization of research. The crisis of the COVID-19 pandemic has elicited a number of unprecedented emergency regulatory responses that aim at achieving a deliberate and well-informed balancing of interests. The goals of these emergency procedures are to reduce practical obstacles, save efforts, resources, and time, and ensure a rigorous ethical assessment of COVID-19-related research protocols.

As a response to these ongoing challenges, many organisations have reorganized their procedures and have adjusted them to the special COVID-19 circumstances. The main aim of these reforms has been to create a fast-track legal environment for the development and testing of effective and safe means (drugs, vaccines, tests) for the treatment, prevention and diagnosis of SARS-CoV-2 infections. Reforming these procedures was essential in order to safeguard that all major public health and privacy ethics principles are well-protected.

Since the beginning of the COVID-19 pandemic, the World Health Organization (WHO) and the Pan American Health Organization (PAHO) have emphasized the moral duty to conduct ethical research in response to the pandemic and have developed operational strategies and guidance on key ethical issues for ethics review and oversight taking into account the lessons learned from past outbreaks.

The urgency related to the pandemic forced many jurisdictions and the EU to introduce expedited review procedures for AI-related research protocols which have also led many data protection authorities to adjust their notification and evaluation procedures to the increased regulatory needs associated with the deployment of novel technological applications. Most European countries have put in place accelerated procedures for the evaluation and authorization of clinical trials related to the management of the pandemic covering also the ethics review process.

At the EU level, the Commission, in its different COVID-19 related Recommendations and Communications has emphasized the need for technologies deployed to fight the pandemic to respect fundamental rights, notably privacy as well as data protection and prevent surveillance and stigmatization. Throughout the pandemic, the European Data Protection Board and various national data protection authorities and ethics committees have underlined the need for all deployed technological solutions to respect human rights and ethical acquis.

In general, despite the involvement of several ethics committees during the deployment of several AI-powered solutions, their normative footprint remained rather weak and their involvement inconsistent and fragmentary. Ethics committee members' lack of familiarity with the technical features and the potential of these technological applications, the limited time frame within which they had to provide an opinion and their overshadowing by data protection authorities and vaccine advisory committees, appear as the main factors that limited their influence and lasting presence during the various stages of technological response to the pandemic.

13.5 Policy Suggestions

As the COVID-19 pandemic illustrates, times of crisis necessitate rapid deployment of new technologies in order to save lives. However, this urgency both makes it more likely that ethical issues and risks will arise, and makes them more challenging to address. Rather than neglecting ethics, we must find ways to address ethical tensions.

If ethical practices can be implemented with urgency (Tzachor et al. 2020), the current crisis could provide an opportunity to drive greater application of AI for societal benefit, and to ensure AI is used responsibly without undermining protection of fundamental values and human rights. For that reason, this chapter is putting forward a series of policy options that could ensure that AI can be safely and beneficially used in the COVID-19 response and beyond.

First of all, AI applications should be deployed only on the basis of clear, transparent criteria with sunset clauses for emergency legislation. Thus, ethical safeguards need to be embedded in all policy decisions that authorize the use of AI for handling various aspects of the pandemic. The incorporation of clauses of this kind could ensure that the deployment of AI systems is conditional to its constant compliance with ethical norms and lead to the framing of a reflexive framework of emergency technology ethics advice. Beyond the introduction of sunset clauses, other safeguards are needed, including purpose limitation, transparency, explainability of the data processing operations and constant monitoring, especially for automated tracing tools. The drafting of these safeguards requires the meaningful involvement of data protection authorities, local and national ethics committees, and AI designers but also their activation in accordance with commonly agreed guidelines. The introduction of special ethical safeguards into the development and deployment procedures has become an essential condition for the use of AI during COVID-19. A regular review of the continued need for the processing of personal data for the purposes of combating the COVID-19 crisis should be performed and appropriate sunset clauses need to be introduced so as to ensure that the processing does not extend beyond what is strictly necessary for those purposes.

The general AI principles adopted in Europe and elsewhere do not seem to offer sufficient guidance in emergency situations. Where certain values are in conflict, there is an urgent need to support the development of standard operating procedures for emergency response ethical review.

Moreover, AI systems should be designed by taking into account the diversity of socio-economic and healthcare settings. Their development and deployment should be accompanied by community engagement, awareness-raising and digital literacy capacity-building actions, given that the automation of several diagnostic and healthcare tasks could challenge the decision-making and autonomy of healthcare providers and patients. At the same time, policy is needed to ensure that AI systems used in the context of the pandemic are transparent, explainable, robust, secure and safe; also, actors involved in their development and use should remain accountable especially when it comes to temporary measures of population control and monitoring. Within this frame, the principle of explicability becomes particularly important for AI-based decisions about treatment and allocation of resources which require improvement in the accuracy and efficacy of AI-based tools related to medical detection and treatment. Strict interpretation of public health legal exemptions could be crucial to ensuring the responsible use of this disruptive technology during public health emergencies.

The capacity of ethics review mechanisms to react promptly and thoroughly to pressing and demanding challenges needs to be strengthened, not only in institutional and legal terms but also in terms of its positioning within the entire ecosystem of policy advice. Governments, providers, and designers must work together to address ethics and human rights concerns at every stage of an AI technology's design, development, and deployment. In the absence of established legal frameworks, policy, or practice standards that specifically guide research ethics review and oversight, it is imperative to acknowledge the need to address gaps in the ethical governance of health emergencies. This may serve as a basis for the development of a treaty framework that will help ethics boards to anticipate and address issues uniquely associated with rapid advances in technological capabilities and novel applications. Acknowledging the need to address gaps in preventing, preparing for, and responding to health emergencies from an ethical perspective would safeguard timely and equitable access to vaccines, therapeutics and diagnostics and ensure the ethically sound deployment of digital technologies.

What the COVID-19 crisis has made clear to many in the field of health data science and governance is the need for coordinated, dedicated data infrastructures and ecosystems for tackling dynamic societal and environmental threats as well as an improved governance of rapid data sharing. Towards this direction, common data reporting and interoperability rules and standards are needed to ensure trusted sharing of useful data in times of crisis. There is also a policy need to encourage multidisciplinary and multi-stakeholder cooperation and data exchange both nationally and internationally by the AI community, medical community, developers and policy makers to formulate the problems, identify relevant data and open datasets, share tools and train models, and facilitate the responsible sharing of medical, molecular, and scientific datasets and models on collaborative platforms to help AI researchers build effective tools for the medical community.

Last, but not least, derogations of human rights, albeit in the interests of the public good must be temporary, and hence exceptional measures taken by governments for the use of AI must be necessary and proportionate. Therefore, restrictions of rights and freedoms that are imposed in an emergency situation—including those implemented through technological surveillance from mobile devices through to drones and surveillance cameras—need to be removed, and data need to be destroyed, as soon as the emergency is over or infringements are no longer proportionate. Preventing AI use from contributing to the establishment of new forms of automated social control, which could persist long after the epidemic subsides, must be addressed in ongoing legislative initiatives on AI at EU level as some AI systems raise concerns about purpose specification and the danger that personal data could be re-used in ways that infringe privacy and other individual rights.

13.6 Concluding Remarks

In the context of the current pandemic, numerous data-collection and location-tracking technological applications have been launched on the basis of emergency laws that involve the temporary suspension of fundamental rights and authorisation of medical devices and vaccines via fast-tracked procedures (Kritikos 2020c).

Based on the analysis above, several conclusions can be drawn that relate both to the technological readiness and the preparedness of the ethical governance structures to meet the ever-increasing challenges that the rapid deployment of a wide range of AI applications has brought to society and to the policy sphere.

Firstly, unlike previous public health crises, this one indicates that technology in itself and in particular AI is not a technological silver bullet that could contain COVID-19 (Heaven 2020) but should serve as a means not only to digitize the main tenets of the public health ecosystem and facilitate the use of health management AI-based tools and also to reinforce the importance of the human factor in the management of public health crises.

Secondly, although the uptake of AI has been limited mostly to certain aspects of the medical and healthcare domains, its use during the pandemic has illustrated its vast potential to play an increasingly critical role in emergency responses. Thirdly, the deployment of AI-powered applications triggers questions about the effects on civil liberties as well as concerns about state authorities maintaining heightened levels of surveillance, even after the pandemic ends (Kritikos 2020c).

Fourthly, the deployment of AI-powered systems that have not been tested previously on a global scale illustrates not only the limitations of the meaningful involvement of ethics governance structures in policy discussions and their rather weak policy impact in the context of this public health emergency but also the general lack of ethical preparedness to provide policy-relevant guidance and introduce ethical safeguards that go beyond the traditional data protection legal requirements.

Moreover, the current pandemic represents an excellent opportunity for policymakers and regulators to develop a new international pandemics technology ethics framework that could respond to the need for timely ethics advice. The continuous adoption of AI ethics guidelines and frameworks worldwide can in fact pave the way for the shaping of a common, robust procedural framework for ethics advice under emergency conditions.

The uptake of AI applications will not only depend on their technical capacities but also on how inclusive, privacy-friendly and human-centered their algorithmic procedures will end up being. In fact, building public trust around AI may be particularly challenging in crisis times, where review timelines need to be significantly reduced, without compromising on ethical and legal principles and guidelines. The deployment of AI for various applications requires a paradigm shift in the way ethical principles are taken into account and ethics review procedures are followed. If methodologies to perform ethics assessments of technological applications under time pressure are developed swiftly, the current crisis could provide an opportunity to deploy AI for societal benefit, and to build public trust in such applications.

Therefore, the management of the risks associated with infectious diseases is likely to remain an ongoing challenge for local, national and global efforts to shape a robust and transparent ethical governance. Towards this direction, it is essential that processes are put in place in advance to better understand potential trade-offs involved in deploying an AI system and acceptable ways to resolve them. In other words, emergency ethics preparedness needs to be seen not only as part of the policy response to the current pandemic but also as part of the ongoing discussions to build an ethics-by-design framework for the domain of AI (Kritikos 2020d).

References

Berditchevskaia, Aleks, and Kathy Peach. 2020. Coronavirus: Seven ways collective intelligence is tackling the pandemic. World Economic Forum. https://www.weforum.org/agenda/2020/03/cor onavirus-seven-ways-collective-intelligence-is-tackling-the-pandemic. Accessed 17 December 2021.

Bullock, Joseph, Alexandra Luccioni, Katherine Hoffmann Pham, Cynthia Sin Nga Lam, and Miguel Luengo-Oroz. 2020. Mapping the landscape of artificial intelligence applications against COVID-19. arXiv preprint. https://arxiv.org/abs/2003.11336. Accessed 17 December 2021.

Heaven, Will Douglas. 2020. AI could help with the next pandemic but not with this one. MIT Technology Review. https://www.technologyreview.com/s/615351/ai-could-help-with-the-next-pandemicbut-not-with-this-one. Accessed 17 December 2021.

Kim, Max S. 2020. South Korea is watching quarantined citizens with a smartphone app. MIT Technology Review. https://www.technologyreview.com/s/615329/coronavirus-south-korea-smartp hone-app-quarantine. Accessed 17 December 2021.

Kritikos, Mihalis. 2020a. What if AI-powered passenger locator forms could help stop the spread of Covid-19? European Parliamentary Research Service At A Glance. https://www.europarl.eur opa.eu/RegData/etudes/ATAG/2020a/656298/EPRS_ATA(2020a)656298_EN.pdf. Accessed 17 December 2021.

Kritikos Mihalis. 2020b. What if we could fight coronavirus with artificial intelligence? European Parliamentary Research Service At A Glance. https://www.europarl.europa.eu/RegData/etudes/ ATAG/2020/641538/EPRS_ATA(2020)641538_EN.pdf. Accessed 17 December 2021.

Kritikos, Mihalis. 2020c. Ten technologies to fight Coronavirus. European Parliament European Parliamentary Research Service. https://www.europarl.europa.eu/RegData/etudes/IDAN/2020b/ 641543/EPRS_IDA(2020b)641543_EN.pdf. Accessed 17 December 2021.

Kritikos, Mihalis. 2020d. What if artificial intelligence in medical imaging could accelerate Covid-19 treatment? European Parliamentary Research Service At A Glance. https://www.europarl.eur opa.eu/RegData/etudes/ATAG/2020c/656333/EPRS_ATA(2020c)656333_EN.pdf. Accessed 17 December 2021.

Luengo-Oroz, Miguel, Katherine Hoffmann Pham, Joseph Bullock, Robert Kirkpatrick, Alexandra Luccioni, Sasha Rubel, Cedric Wachholz, Moez Chakchouk, Phillippa Biggs, Tim Nguyen, Tina Purnat, and Bernardo Mariano. 2020, Artificial intelligence cooperation to support the global response to COVID-19. *Nature Machine Intelligence* 2: 295–297.

Malgieri, Gianclaudio. 2020. Data Protection and Research: A vital challenge in the era of COVID-19 pandemic. *Computer Law & Security Review* 37: 105431. https://doi.org/10.2139/ssrn.358 0179.

McCall, Becky. 2020. COVID-19 and artificial intelligence: Protecting health-care workers and curbing the spread. *Lancet Digital Health* 2(4): 166–167. https://doi.org/10.1016/S2589-750 0(20)30054-6.

Tang, Bowen, Fengming He, Dongpeng Liu, Meijuan Fang, Zhen Wu, and Dong Xu. 2020. AI-aided design of novel targeted covalent inhibitors against SARSCoV-2. bioRxiv preprint. https://doi. org/10.1101/2020.03.03.972133v1. Accessed 17 December 2021.

Tzachor, Asaf, Jess Whittlestone, Lalitha Sundaram, and Seán Ó hÉigeartaigh. 2020. Artificial intelligence in a crisis needs ethics with urgency. *Nature Machine Intelligence* 2(7): 365–366.

Van der Schaar, Mihaela, Ahmed M. Alaa, Andres Floto, Alexander Gimson, Stefan Scholtes, Angela Wood, Eoin McKinney, Daniel Jarrett, Pietro Lio, and Ari Ercole. 2020. How artificial intelligence and machine learning can help healthcare systems respond to COVID-19. *Machine Learning*.https://doi.org/10.1007/s10994-020-05928-x.

Chapter 14
Automated Justice: Issues, Benefits and Risks in the Use of Artificial Intelligence and Its Algorithms in Access to Justice and Law Enforcement

Caroline Gans-Combe

Abstract The use of artificial intelligence (AI) in the field of law has generated many hopes. Some have seen it as a way of relieving courts' congestion, facilitating investigations, and making sentences for certain offences more consistent—and therefore fairer. But while it is true that the work of investigators and judges can be facilitated by these tools, particularly in terms of finding evidence during the investigative process, or preparing legal summaries, the panorama of current uses is far from rosy, as it often clashes with the reality of field usage and raises serious questions regarding human rights. This chapter will use the Robodebt Case to explore some of the problems with introducing automation into legal systems with little human oversight. AI—especially if it is poorly designed—has biases in its data and learning pathways which need to be corrected. The infrastructures that carry these tools may fail, introducing novel bias. All these elements are poorly understood by the legal world and can lead to misuse. In this context, there is a need to identify both the users of AI in the area of law and the uses made of it, as well as a need for transparency, the rules and contours of which have yet to be established.

Keywords Artificial intelligence · Law enforcement · Judicial system · Evidence gathering · Sentencing · Adversarial right · Automation · Enquiries · Overcollection

When Deanna Amato had her tax deductions withheld by Centrelink in 2019—a service of the Australian government's Income Compliance Program, responsible at the time for, among other things, the recovery of social security overpayments—she had no idea that this was one of the many erroneous outputs of an automated legal decision-making software. The so-called Robodebt case involved hundreds of thousands of Australians being issued automated reports that they owed money to the Australian welfare system. It was later acknowledged that the use of inadequate

C. Gans-Combe (✉)
Inseec Business School, Head of Structured Research, Omnes Education Research Center, Paris, France
e-mail: cganscombe@omneseducation.com

© The Author(s) 2022
D. O'Mathúna and R. Iphofen (eds.), *Ethics, Integrity and Policymaking*, Research Ethics Forum 9, https://doi.org/10.1007/978-3-031-15746-2_14

data associated with a rogue algorithmic practice resulted in the Australian Government sending out more than 400,000 requests for refunds of non-existent social overpayments (Bennett 2019).

This so-called "Robodebt" case demonstrated that the uncontrolled use of artificial intelligence and machine learning tools for decision-making purposes with legal impacts is far from mature, notwithstanding the billions of dollars in revenue already generated annually by these types of tools (Alston 2019).

The Robodebt case: The Robodebt scheme, also known as the Centrelink debt recovery program, ran between 2015 and November 2019. Using comparison algorithms, Centrelink, an Australian social security state agency, matched the average annual tax rates and tax payments of tax deduction recipients with their actual fortnightly tax returns. If a difference in amount was found in favour of the social security administration, the algorithm systematically concluded that there was an error in the declaration and automatically launched a recovery procedure. In effect, welfare recipients were assumed to owe money until they could prove otherwise. Even worse, Centrelink issued a debt notice based on averaged Australian Taxation Office (ATO) information alone and applied a 10% penalty. Centrelink did not use its information-gathering powers to contact the concerned taxpayer's employers or banks to provide details of actual earnings for the relevant fortnights to determine whether the taxpayer actually owed the automated debt calculation. When exposed through the Amato case, the proceeding resulted in a large class-action suit, exposing a massive failure of public administration as the government unlawfully raised $1.76 billion in debts against 443,000 people. During that time, the Australian government had also pursued about 381,000 people, unlawfully recovering $751 million, including through private debt collectors. In court, the Australian Government conceded that the averaging process using ATO income data to calculate all Robodebt was unlawful.

Thus, the illusion that administrative or legal procedures can be facilitated or accelerated clashes with the reality of field usage, and raises serious questions regarding human rights (Langford 2020), notwithstanding the strong impacts on involved or concerned parties and an even more significant effect on vulnerable populations (Carney 2020).

In this context, this chapter has three objectives:

- To identify the types of cases concerned by these situations to propose perimeters of vigilance as well as to identify the critical paths leading to potential errors.
- To identify (through the different cases raised in existing publications) the elements of technological design that can lead to the scandals and biases mentioned above: the "glitches" in the sense of Meunier et al. (2019).

– To suggest some good practices to help the supporters of this type of solution to prosper without damaging public liberties, the rights of the citizens or the possibilities of unbiased access to law and justice.

14.1 Where and How the Automation of Legal Acts Takes Place

The example of "Robodebt" has made it possible to highlight that the use of algorithms in processes with legal impacts is not limited to the courts of justice. Artificial intelligence (AI) is the set of theories and techniques implemented to create machines capable of simulating human intelligence in its neural architecture for various uses and in various fields. It combines a set of technological tools (deep learning, structured or unstructured predictive analysis, data) at the origin of methods for solving problems with high logical and/or algorithmic complexity. There are therefore many uses open to AI (support, data collection, decision making, learning, prediction), which can be found in what is known today as LegalTech, i.e. the involvement of technology in developing, proposing or providing products or services related to law and justice. The LegalTech market will be worth more than US$25 billion by 2025, with US$6.37 billion in the European market alone (Alsop et al. 2020).

It, therefore, seems useful, as a preliminary step, to propose a mapping of the concerned domains. The mapping proposed in this chapter is matrix-based. First, it is divided into two branches, the branch where the action of algorithms replaces the judge and the branch where the action of algorithms supports the judge, each of them having its own justifications and operationality, and raising questions about legality, the legal system, public liberties and even efficiency. Finally, it is grouped in a transverse questioning that covers what could be called predictive or prophetic law: the data coming from both the results of the decision support and the positive actions of substitutions to the judge (for example, which automated decisions are more likely to be appealed) being themselves concatenated to permanently reformulate the perimeter and the distribution of the elements of the matrix (Fig. 14.1: The distinctive branches of AI use in the field of law and justice).

Today the substitution—at least the one perceived by the simple citizen—often covers only subjects of first instance law (parking fines, speeding tickets, tax or social deductions), but tomorrow we can imagine a tightening of practices limiting the appeal procedures or making them as complex as possible to avoid the occurrence of such disputes. The practical result would be the use of algorithms to distance the citizen from the law or from the exercise of his rights. The appeal of an automated decision is indeed quite complex, especially to access a human explaining clearly the procedures to follow (and even when he is trained to do so). In the Robodebt case, the Centrelink service at the origin of the scandal had such a long waiting time (more than 15 min online) to access a call center of untrained agents, that the only recourse for the citizens was a class action suit which still has a devastating impact both financially and in terms of image for the company, notwithstanding the intervention of many

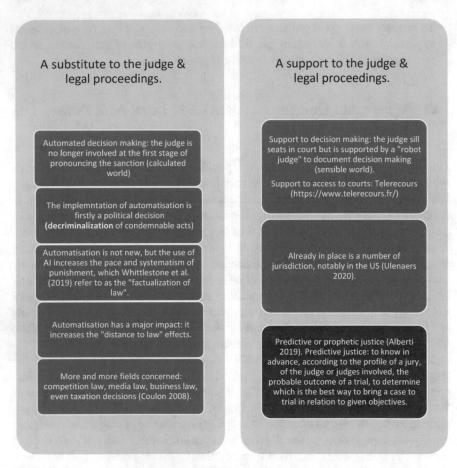

Fig. 14.1 The distinctive branches of "AI uses" in the field of law and justice

spin doctors to try to redress the situation (Towell 2017). Indeed, the proceedings, some of which are still ongoing, have so far cost the Australian state and the social security administration a total of A$1.8 billion.

The substitution of judges by other legal operators, such as arbitrators or mediators, called alternative disputes resolutions (ADR), is becoming increasingly common, in business or family law for example. There is thus a habit of differentiated practices that is taking root in society (Ferrand 2015).

At the same time, the interference of digital technologies in the legal process is not limited to the use of artificial intelligence (Ulenaers 2020). It is an older and broader issue (Stranieri et al. 1999) than the question underlying the intrusion of this new approach into the legal world or in the service of the legal ecosystem. Therefore, the issues raised are both non-specific and specific to AI. All the subjects to be analyzed below related to access to law, and to the respect of the adversarial process, are non-specific inasmuch as they relate to automation as to AI, whereas AI raises specific issues in the approaches related to network and data architectures, to the quality of the data and especially its neutrality. These new uses (deep learning, etc.) increase the paradox between the expectation of neutrality with regard to the judge's decision and the respect for public liberties.

14.1.1   Why Substitute Judges with Algorithmic/Automated Operations?

The substituting of judges with algorithms has been justified by the need to relieve overloaded courts of justice. Political actors on all sides have been trying to do this since access to the law was considered a fundamental right during the Enlightenment (Gray 2008).

Indeed, access to the judge to settle disputes with the constituted bodies (police, state, etc.) grew very quickly as people developed an expectation for a justice system that was autonomous from political actors (Bell et al. 2004), and that could be considered neutral. However, since the beginning of this century, justice, like the political-administrative ecosystem that is part of the rule of law, is in crisis (Stoett 2019). It suffers from a triple conflict between expectations, means and legitimacy (Fig. 14.2: The three tensions facing the judiciary).

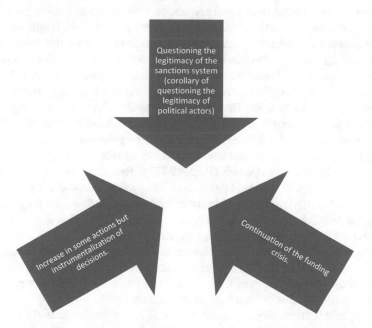

Fig. 14.2   The three tensions facing the judiciary

Expectations: if recourse to depenalization—i.e. the exclusion of certain disputes from the scope of the first instance judge—has had a definite effect on the volume of cases to be tried (we will come back to this in detail below), the contestation of the administration's actions and decisions in courts is at best stable, and at worst rising sharply, including in member countries where the rule of law is undermined.

Means: if the financial means are globally increasing, they remain quite scarce compared to the populations concerned: in this respect, Switzerland (a non-EU member state) is by far the European country that invests the most money per inhabitant in its judicial system. With an expenditure of €220.6 per inhabitant in 2018, well ahead of Luxembourg (€163.5) and Germany (€131.2). The three least well-endowed states within the European Union are Lithuania (€41.5 per inhabitant), Bulgaria (€42.3) and Romania (€42.6). All other EU members fall in between (European Commission 2021).

Legitimacy: the imperative of judicial neutrality (Ellis 2018) has been undermined on the one hand by the instrumentalization of the processes of appointing magistrates by politics, and on the other hand by the politically marked decisions that have quite naturally followed (Delsol 2021).

The impact of this probing of the legitimacy of decisions taken by judges has been reinforced by the relatively continuous questioning by whole segments of the European population—since the beginning of the COVID-19 crisis—of the legitimacy of elected decision-makers. When these actors have not demonstrated what Parviainen et al. (2021) have called "Epistemic Humility", problems arise. Instead, they present to the public their sometimes biased certainties. "When the law obliterates itself at the top, everything becomes permitted," Jean Pierre Delsol (2021) rightly tells us.

To *a request for neutrality,* the public actors answered by the automation of certain decision-making. This was based on the following presupposition: A decision made by an automated device would not be influenced by humans and would be in compliance with the law. This is true, but a decision that is legal at a given time does not imply that it is right or fair (Barocas and Hardt 2017), nor that this legality will remain over time. History is replete with the instrumentalization of the rule of law for political purposes—is it worth recalling the sinister legalism of the Nazis who made the Final Solution legal under the laws of the time and the country, of which Hanna Arendt has painted a vivid picture (Poizat 2017)? Robodebt, or the fines imposed on drivers who respect the law, in this case, the speed limits—due to a change in legislation not carried over in time in the machines—underlines the fragility of the assumption that the machine can't go wrong. Yet that assumption is still supported by many public actors in Europe (Pasquale 2019).

These are the first limits to legal automation: the hiatus between the legality of the sanction and the reality of the infringement. Just because an offence has been found by a machine does not mean that it is genuine or meaningful from a legal point of view. The context is just as important as the offence itself.

The appetite for neutrality appears therefore as one of the elements of the observed tendency to automate judicial proceedings. Other more fundamental intentions are added to this. It will be recalled that the European Union measures the legal performance of each member country according to three criteria (European Commission 2021):

- **Efficiency**, which focuses on indicators such as the length of proceedings, the rate of variation of the stock of pending cases and the number of pending cases.
- **Quality**, which highlights indicators related to accessibility, such as legal aid and court fees, training, budget, human resources, and digitization.
- **Independence**, which focuses on indicators relating to the perception of the independence of justice by the general public and businesses, guarantees concerning judges and guarantees concerning the functioning of national prosecution offices.

14.2   Problems Raised by the Substitution of Automation for the Judge

Admittedly, as indicated in the latest iteration of the Council of Europe's European Commission for the Efficiency of Justice (CEPEJ 2020a), automation makes it possible to reduce the response time to a legal problem, and thus the congestion of the courts, especially when they deal with only relatively low-value disputes. But this practice poses serious problems as regards the rule of law because:

a. this is problematic in terms of respecting the principle of adversarial proceedings, which is a positive right recognized both by Article 47 of the Charter of Fundamental Rights of the European Union and by Article 6 of the European Convention on Human Rights.
b. it requires the removal from the control of the judge (for the benefit of administrations often under the tutelage of the Executive) a whole part of the societal activity by decriminalizing certain facts (Croze 2017).
c. it condemns more than it exonerates. The automation is systematically incriminating because it is only interested in the potential offender, but it can be wrong (we have seen this with the problems of speeding or parking tickets as well as Robodebt). The burden of proof is then on the potential offender, who must prove that he was not at fault, which is complex, since he may not have legal training (Maurel 2019). The wrongdoing is then converted into a sanction without measure or understanding of the ecosystem. As such, the process breaks the social dimension of justice by reducing it to a mere decision. Justice is fundamentally a process, and trials, as they unfold, contribute to the acceptance of sentences.
d. it raises questions about access to the law and corrective procedures in the event of a challenge to the ultimate decision.

It should be recalled that the European Commission itself, in order to deny access to documents and elements of internal procedures, hides behind the notion of "space to think". The legal contours here are vague, even though the principle is expressly condemned by the Court of Justice of the European Communities (Judgement of the General Court (Seventh Chamber, Extended Composition) of 22 March 2018 in case

T-540/15 De Capitani / Parliament) on the grounds that an EU decision cannot be opposed to a citizen on the basis of elements to which he or she has not had access (Hillebrandt and Novak 2016). "It would violate an elementary principle of law to base a judicial decision on facts and documents of which the parties or any of them have not been able to take notice and on which they have therefore not been able to adopt a position" (Judgment of the Court of 22 March 1961.—Société nouvelle des usines de Pontlieue—Aciéries du Temple (S.N.U.P.A.T.) v High Authority of the European Coal and Steel Community.—Joined cases 42 and 49/59).

The principle of adversarial proceedings has been consecrated as a general principle of law by most of the supreme national jurisdictions in European countries (Ferrand 2000) and is included in Article 6 §1 of the European Convention for the Protection of Human Rights (CESDH). Even if this principle seems to apply to only the judge according to the drafting of the aforementioned Article 16, such is not the case since all the legal actors are also debtors of the respect of the contradictory. The European Court of Human Rights (ECHR) stated this in its Mantovanelli v. France judgment (ECHR, March 18, 1997, no. 21497/93). In this case, the applicants challenged the enforceability of the expert report on the grounds that the conclusions of the legal expert were based on elements that had been communicated to them without respecting the adversarial process.

The adversarial principle guarantees that the parties will not be judged without having been heard, or at least called. A person who has not been informed of the proceedings against him or her has certain guarantees, both in terms of the remedies available and the enforcement of the decision. The principle of adversarial proceedings guarantees each party the right to be informed of the arguments of fact, law and evidence upon which it will be judged. The various participants in the trial must therefore be loyal and diligent in communicating their documents and conclusions. Any element produced in court must be able to be debated and must therefore be communicated to the opponent.

The judge himself is required to respect the adversarial principle. For example, when he considers raising a legal argument of his own, he must give the parties the opportunity to explain this point, otherwise, he will not be able to use it in his decision. In the Mantovanelli v. France judgment (ECHR, March 18, 1997, no. 21497/93), the ECHR recalled that with the principle of adversarial proceedings, "the essential thing is that the parties are able to participate adequately in the proceedings before the 'court'." None of this is possible in the case of automated decisions because the latter precede the debate, not follow it.

There is thus potentially a pronouncement of the sanction "in abstentia", based on exogenous mechanical elements (the speed is x and such and such a driver has exceeded it by y) without the litigant having any means of ex-ante contradiction. The context of non-compliance with a law is not addressed: should a driver be convicted of speeding when he could potentially be transporting a dying COVID-19 patient to the hospital? A judge would admit the (so-called) mitigating circumstance and probably limit the impact of a conviction to the pedagogical understanding that not respecting road safety constitutes a danger. The machine will automatically condemn, and make the person pay a fine before allowing the launching of a possibly contradictory procedure. A deposit is often compulsory to contest the case, which restricts access to the justice system for the poorest people who do not have the means to block the funds or to mobilize the means to take legal action.

An automation process, or an AI that would respect this principle, has yet to be invented. Therefore, the solution currently found is the depenalization of certain situations. "Legal depenalization" covers two hypotheses. Firstly, it can consist of a downgrading of a given behaviour within the penal system: a crime becomes a misdemeanour; a misdemeanour becomes a contravention. The behaviour remains prohibited but punished less severely. Secondly, depenalization can also consist in taking a behaviour out of criminal law and into another legal sphere: civil law, administrative law, etc. (Jaafari 2016). The said conduct is still prohibited, but it will be sanctioned by another authority such as an alternate court circuit, or by an independent administrative authority such as the Competition Authority in France (financial sanction: Coulon 2008). Depenalization is frequently used to transform road traffic offences into simple contraventions (Fallery 2019).

Since the object is no longer the domain of the judge but of an administrative authority, not only does automation become possible but the nature of recourse to the judge is displaced: it is no longer a question of validating the existence or not of a fault but of arbitrating between two interpretations of a fact by two actors who are opposed to each other and whose relations are necessarily unbalanced (Ellis 2018). It is no longer the triptych 'law—judge—citizen' that meets but the triptych 'citizen—administration—law' arbitrated by the judge. The law is set by the administrative authority and the judge must only validate the adequate interpretation. The question put to the court is no longer, 'is there fault therefore sanction?', but, 'is the sanction valid with regard to the offence?'.

In this sense, automation transforms profoundly and durably the balance of the social interactions between litigants and justice, at the risk perhaps of upsetting such interchanges. Indeed, in this automatic response, there is a break between cause and effect, and the person subject to trial who has not been confronted with justice will probably find it difficult to understand what he or she is accused of, and therefore to accept the sentence (Bathaee 2017). This is another element feeding the crisis of confidence that citizens have towards their institutions (Guggeis 2020).

In this context, artificial intelligence—and deep learning—is one more tool at the service of an already advanced process. It is not so much the process of automation that is being questioned, but how the architecture of AI and associated technologies impact existing automation tools by modifying them, even though the legal questions they raise have hardly been resolved.

This inquiry makes sense when we look at the second branch of our mapping of automation in the field of justice (Fig. 14.1): the support provided to the judge and to the judicial process.

14.3 Automation as a Support to the judge's Decision or as a Procedural Assistant

Another area where automation is nowadays omnipresent is judicial decision support. The issue here is far more critical, as it is not limited to justice alone, but also to investigative procedures; in other words, to law enforcement.

The Council of Europe has since 2018 deployed an ethical charter of good practice in the use of AI in legal proceedings and/or as an investigative tool. This doctrinal approach rather than positive law is to be regretted, as it singularly weakens the scope of this publication, which therefore has no binding value (Hyde 2019).

Legal proceedings, especially in criminal matters, call for much information from various sources and of various kinds. The role of AI in legal matters (Prakken and Sartor 2002) is to classify, link and integrate them without omitting any elements. With this support, the investigator and/or the magistrate can view, analyze and compare more documents in an increasingly voluminous and complex file.

AI is a complex set of means likely to endow computer systems with cognitive capacities in order to analyze data in large quantities, with statistical and probabilistic tools and with algorithms that classify, value and confront these sets.

Obviously, there are access limitations related to confidentiality, security or anonymization. Nevertheless, these data can naturally be coupled with other data, which may or may not be freely accessible, in order to constitute resource bases for end-users capable of linking, classifying, contextualizing and cross-referencing them. This allows finer information, with a better granularity, to be calculated or extrapolated than exists in their sources.

In this complex context, two "applications typologies" exist: expert systems and machine learning. In expert systems, the tool is taught by providing it with examples; in machine learning, the tool is asked to find, among the data it has access to, what is likely to be of interest. Expert systems are built on explanatory models to which parameters must be associated to establish one or several results. Machine learning algorithms are used in situations where a mechanistic approach not enhanced by the performance of algorithms is to be excluded.

Hence, machine learning will aim to develop a realistic correlation model between predictive variables (input data) and target variables (results). To do this, machine learning relies on a set of statistical tools and computer algorithms automating the construction of a prediction function (Singh et al. 2007).

An expert system is a tool capable of replicating the cognitive mechanisms of a human expert. For example, it could be software capable of answering questions, by reasoning from known facts and rules. It has 3 parts: a fact base, a rule base and an inference engine: a "thinking machine" (Ross 1933). *The inference engine can use facts and rules to induce further facts until it finds the answer to the given "expert query".*

Machine learning uses an inductive approach to build a mathematical model from data, including many variables that are not known in advance. The parameters are configured as they are learned in a training phase, which uses training data sets to find and classify links. Designers chose different machine learning methods depending on the nature of the task at hand.

Expert systems rely on mathematically constructed logic and use deductive reasoning. As such, they are considered the first level of what constitutes Artificial Intelligence. Despite their performance in many fields, the choices deduced by the algorithms are difficult to explain in simple terms. This difficulty is increased by the paradigm shift introduced by deep learning. Thus, the choice of the learning technique used, the ethics of design, the absence of bias and the absolute necessity of being able to explain the arguments that allowed the tool to make a particular decision are all prohibitive elements in the initial construction of these support tools. This is where the problems arise (Whittlestone et al. 2019).

Several emblematic cases can be mentioned:

14.3.1 Easing Access to Law Enforcement and Filing

The deployment of automation and AI speeds up how files are processed, sorted, and considered, contributing to access to the law. Professionals see their workload reduced by tools like "telerecours" (facilitation of procedures reserved for legal professionals), while other instruments bring citizens closer to law enforcement authorities, notably through automated complaint tools (for example, with cyber-crimes: https://www.europol.europa.eu/report-a-crime/report-cybercrime-online).

14.3.2 Solving Criminal Cases: Artificial Intelligence and Judicial Investigation

During an investigation, data are linked together with observations of a crime scene or misdemeanour. In a few years, this has gone from sketches to 3D extrapolations which include the statements of traces and various objects whose utility for a file is not necessarily established at the very beginning of the enquiry. We are in the middle of over-collection of declarations, testimonies, and hearings which often constitute the first step in the search for contradictions or verifications of facts. However, this collection is a prerequisite for the establishment of what is known as the index value, i.e. the interest and justification of the samples. If AI arrives to accomplish classification (and thus of operational enhancement through the construction of logical links), cross-checking and connecting facts and clues in the judicial files, the expectation is that the truth will be exposed in the trial. For this, various methodologies are used ranging from systematic automation (such as for recognition of people or objects), the establishment of models of existing relationships between information (so-called relational links), the detection of inconsistencies, for example between testimonies using semantic tools (Keyvanpour et al. 2011). All this information is made available to the investigator or the judge without any filter and often without him understanding its full power and scope. Of course, the demonstration of the truth implies authorizing a certain form of exploitation of mass data but ignores ethical questions about over-collection, post-processing, extensive cross-referencing, etc. If the matching work is well understood and structured, the question of false positives remains open. The balance between revealing the truth and considerable means of investigation must be raised. For if these practices are undeniably useful, they require an objective and strong framework. Otherwise, they risk becoming social scoring or the involvement of innocent third parties whose only fault will have been to be virtually identified as having a link with a person of interest.

In this sense, the data collected is central, but also, the data architecture, particularly about the links established. It is certainly necessary to control the algorithms, their level of transparency, but probably also the objectives given to them, because if not done, the power of AI could be misused. For example, tools could anticipate jury decisions by analyzing their profiles (especially in the United States, where contradictory opinions are expressed, including during jury selection). This differs from France, where juries are drawn by lot from citizens, and are used less and less in favour of professional judges. Another example could be the anticipation of judges' decisions by analyzing their pronouncements. Depending on the analytical results, legal strategies may evolve where some litigants may request a change of jury or of location, while others will not have this possibility (Thagard 2004). Similarly, the use of AI attacks the integrity of the evidence by restricting the judge's choice over the validity of the expert opinions provided (Katz 2014). Such examples call for the greatest caution in weighing the contributions of this type of tool to the judicial world.

14.3.3 Predictive or Prophetic Justice

We must also mention areas that carry the most fear and fantasy about automation: predictive or prophetic justice (Queudot and Meurs 2018). This involves predicting the future of a legal action in order to anticipate it (which is sometimes presented as risk management) or to harmonise the scope of sanctions according to given offences/crimes. In addition to the ethical and fairness issues, experiments conducted in France and Europe (Aguzzi 2020) have so far shown reasoning biases leading to aberrant results. The use of algorithms for predictions could flout the principle of sentences in criminal matters and reproduce or reinforce inequalities.

This raises other issues. Firstly, the operation of existing algorithms remains in the hands of their designers due to business secrecy (Singh et al. 2021). Transparency about their design is highly limited, even though justice actors have embryonic expertise to evaluate them. Secondly, because algorithms ignore the possible interpretation of texts and the social context of judgements, the use of AI in justice entails a risk of standardising legal decisions.

14.4 Errors and Risks of the Interference of Artificial Intelligence in Legal Procedures: Integrating the Gap Between the Calculated World and the Sensible World

Meunier et al. (2019) propose an innovative approach extending to algorithms the phenomena of malfunctions affecting electrical systems, machines, software and interfaces (Berti-Equille et al. 2011). The aim is to identify the "bias zones" into which legal algorithms can fall, due to either structural errors or faulty assumptions. The goal is to detect when the algorithm fails either by going beyond the expectations of its designer or deviating from or misinterpreting its underlying assumptions. As AI learns from its own actions, it only takes one faulty element for the whole process to become biased. This could generate false positives which have little impact when it comes to not authorising a payment, but which, when applied to justice, can have otherwise serious effects.

With the progressive "datafication" of all human acts, data is at the heart of the problem. Are the algorithmic biases that often appear during the implementation of this type of process linked to the data collected, to the nature of the data collected, or to the methodologies for using the data? In other words, is it a question of the quality of the data, of the use of the data, or both?

This question was not born with AI. This goes back to the early days of cybernetics—the science of human government—which led people to believe that a society 'steered and managed by machines' would help humans avoid repeating the futile and bloody conflicts of history (Bateson 1972). This assumption ignored that behind the machines there were always humans, and they could only structure the machines according to their own conditioning or culture, reproducing or even reinforcing existing societal inequalities. Thus, many of the indicators that underpin medical decision-making and yet are used every day are—despite themselves—racialised (Cerdeña et al. 2020). There is no reason why justice and its automations should escape this problem (O'Neil 2016). AI gives greater resonance to these biases: it sorts and directs the choices of social actors, including judges, helps them make decisions, assigns indicators of recidivism, and supports recruitment processes. However, the points of vigilance that should be present at all levels of data collection, construction and interpretation are absent. Only the method of calculation and its efficiency or non-efficiency are addressed.

However, O'Neil, like other authors (Richard 2018), has faced much criticism, on the grounds that new algorithms would smooth out old biases until a form of quasi-automated 'algorithmic fairness' was achieved, with differences that would be measurable using dedicated indicators (Chadli et al. 2021). In other words, to improve technology, more technology is needed.

The question of bias is thus answered by calculated answers, even though the bodies of data that feed these systems remain imbued with pre-existing structural inequalities. Thus, algorithmic systems are trained on data that correspond to categorisations that have been the subject of very human choices. AI has not created labels like "individual at high risk of recidivism" or "having a cardiovascular risk".

Ensuring a neutral reading of data does not guarantee its quality or accuracy. If the algorithm notices a bias in a body of data, it should refrain from using this source or correct the biased features, i.e. be able to look critically at its data source. Although data research has taken up the subject (Chereni et al. 2020), tools using AI for decision-making purposes are already being deployed on a large scale. Predictive policing, too, works with "manipulated" data because it relies on information about decades of past convictions without considering that these themselves may be the result of past societal biases (Noriega 2020). The same scenario can be found for algorithms used in the justice sector to detect the risk of recidivism (and thus possibly increase sentences). These are known to be largely unfavourable to certain populations. Even when smoothing out the first instance biases, Cyclic Redundant Coding (CRC) practices dedicated to the detection of errors in databases make it possible to recover traits by verifying other typologies of (socio-demographic) indicators that illustrate membership of given groups in the population. Information can be unintentionally modified during its transmission or storage in memory. Codes must therefore be used to detect or even correct errors due to these modifications. These codes cover more information than that strictly necessary to encode the information. To 'm' data bits, we add 'k' control bits. This means that $n = m + k$ bits will be transmitted or stored in memory. These are known as redundant codes (Ntoutsi et al. 2020). Currently, some methodologies exist to support choices that are free from influences linked to the socio-historical context and economic imperatives. Indeed, even before tackling the technical part, ethical issues, such as the protection of people and their rights, must be integrated into the design of AI processes, as this will influence their architecture and the so-called "learning model" (supervised or unsupervised). In a supervised model, the training data is mastered by the designers who statistically structured the concerned dataset (this is called "data prep") to avoid discrepancies (adequate population sizes and distributions). In an unsupervised model, the neural network itself detects bias. The network must learn to identify what is or can be a bias. The second important focus must be on the training dataset, the information used to teach the network how to behave. Usually, this is part of the global dataset used. If this dataset is biased (statistically not sound), the training will suffer the same failures. As such, a dataset including certain labels (race consideration for example) should not be used. This operation must be done with very special care at the three levels of data processing (pre -, in- and post), and all data that might introduce bias should be excluded in this very moment. Finally, a neural network is never fully trained. Periodic checks for bias in the results are important. AI tools can lose efficiency and performance over time, which, in the case of automated court decisions, could have serious societal impacts. Finally, and often forgotten, AI infrastructure is just as fundamental as the data itself. Collections made in real-time (e.g. stock market prices) can suffer from delays in their injection time into the processes, computers can break down, and, in the end, each grain of sand can bias the outputs.

The potential fallibility of AI's predictability is precisely the reason for creating points of vigilance. The choices that prejudge the design of the tools deployed today actually raise questions that are more ethical than technical. These considerations can be reconsidered by abandoning the idea that society would be powerless in the face of AI's opaque functioning. The tools currently deployed in the field of justice are far from neutral. To ensure the implementation of balanced or neutralised algorithms, three levels of intervention must be considered:

- The data
- The data integrity test
- The calculation, i.e. the algorithm.

These three layers are well known and understood on an individual basis by deep learning domain specialists. We know that ethical AI can be deployed; the only obstacle is the societal will to do so.

14.5 Recommendations by Way of Conclusion

In applying AI to the judicial and law enforcement domains, the question of the promoters of these processes arises. In concrete terms, this amounts to questioning the decision-making power in the field, both in terms of the structure and the reasons inherent to deploying this type of tool.

In law and justice, most people point to their multiple advantages. LegalTech advocates keep repeating that by automating certain tasks, AI would lighten the daily lives of judges and lawyers by relieving them of certain administrative constraints. Judges could also rely on AI for decision support, while lawyers would refine their strategies thanks to the case analyses proposed by AI. As for litigants, the creation of databases from court decisions would give them access to a real legal library. They could see the cost of their proceedings fall due to simplified management, and the time taken to appear in court would decrease.

The problem is that while the costs of implementation are known, the benefits, both operational and financial, for stakeholders other than the promoters of these tools remain unclear (Tung 2019). For example, although the potential financial savings from these deployments are frequently discussed (Rigano 2019), statistics on the reality of these gains are sorely lacking. The cost/benefit trade-off should be reviewed in the light of transparent economic impact studies, as it is not certain that systematisation in this area would be genuinely efficient at optimising the resource use, notably public judicial funds. Regardless, if it seems that AI would improve support for the legal process, it is unclear whether it can be considered a tool for justice in the full sense of the word at present (Wachter et al. 2021).

Certainly, AI could have macroeconomic effects (Mateu and Pluchart 2019). Political and institutional support for LegalTech actors as a well-thought-out tool for international leadership can be agreed upon. This would be a continuation of the multi-secular struggle of legal systems around the world (Ogus 1999). But questions remain as to whether these reasons are of sufficient importance to the general interest to justify and continue supporting technical arbitrations that are known to be biased (Pasquale 2020).

By combining the recommendations of the EU strategy for AI (Act, A. I. EUR-Lex-52021PC0206, 2021), especially point 3.5 on fundamental rights, the institutional studies carried out on this subject (Spajosevic et al. 2020), the analyses of the Council of Europe (CEPEJ 2020b), and the visions of major specialists in the field (Pasquale 2020; O'Neil 2016), certain features of a broad response to the problems mentioned above are emerging. They can be summarised in four points, all of which are based on a logic of 'guaranteed transparency' of systems.

A—Knowledge of the production triptych: the promoter/financier, the designer, the developer

An AI is only a tool that will answer a given question. The more societal the question, the more neutral the AI must be in its learning to be accepted. This implies moderation operations that have yet to be deployed, specifically to avoid what is called "false positives" As a reminder, a false positive is the Bayesian result of making a decision in a two-choice situation that is declared positive when it is actually negative. The outcome may be the result of a hypothesis test, an automatic classification algorithm, or even an arbitrary choice. However, if false positives are tolerable in terms of payment by bank card (after all, it can prevent compulsive purchases), it is unacceptable in terms of justice because it attacks the very foundations of equality, and therefore the balance of our societies. Destroying the balance amounts to destroying all confidence in social systems that are already under attack from populists.

Each AI deployed in the legal field, and therefore likely to become a tool for generating evidence, should have its promoters and developers identified so that the results of this type of activity can be integrated into the adversarial process in the same way as other types of evidence. Without falling into any kind of naivety, calculated evidence should be challenged in the same way as observed or recorded evidence.

B—Knowledge of the essential characteristics of the algorithms

The nature of information processing (supervised or unsupervised learning), and of the associated processes of moderation, whether human or calculated (so-called 'neutralising' bias), should be made public if only to demonstrate their existence.

C—Knowledge of the sources, nature and architecture of the data used to train the algorithms

Whether data is structured or unstructured, and in particular the so-called data-prep processes, should be made clear. This would make it possible to test the quality of the data and therefore the reliability of the foundations of the AI.

D—Knowledge of uses to avoid unanticipated uses

Any technology can be misused. It is not a question, as some suggest, of issuing authorisations for use, but of knowing who uses this type of tool and why.

All this information could be deposited in a supra-national registry (perhaps carried out by the EU) in return for which applicants would be granted rights or certificates of use as suggested by the CEPEJ in its feasibility study (CEPEJ 2020c). Once this knowledge ecosystem has been established, the possible deployment and further uses of an algorithmic approach to justice can be imagined, ensuring that artificial intelligence is put to the service of all.

References

Act, A.I. 2021. Proposal for a regulation of the European Parliament and the Council laying down harmonised rules on Artificial Intelligence (Artificial Intelligence Act) and amending certain Union legislative acts. *EUR-Lex-52021PC0206*. https://eur-lex.europa.eu/legal-content/EN/HIS/?uri=CELEX:52021PC0206. Accessed 19 December 2021.

Alston, P. 2019. Digital technology, social protection and human rights: Report. OHCHR. https://www.ohchr.org/EN/Issues/Poverty/Pages/DigitalTechnology.aspx. Accessed 17 May 2021.

Alsop, T., S. Calio, and P. Greis. 2020. LEGAL TECH: A Statista dossier on the worldwide Legal Tech market. https://www.statista.com/study/84775/legal-tech. Accessed 4 December 2022.

Aguzzi, C. 2020. Le juge et l'intelligence artificielle: La perspective d'une justice rendue par la machine. *Annuaire International De Justice Constitutionnelle* 35 (2019): 621–636.

Barocas, S., and M. Hardt. 2017. NIPS tutorial on fairness in machine learning. https://fairmlbook.org/tutorial1.html. Accessed 4 December 2022.

Bateson, G. 1972. From Versailles to cybernetics. In *Steps to an Ecology of Mind*, 477–485. London: Jason Aronson, Inc.

Bathaee, Y. 2017. The artificial intelligence black box and the failure of intent and causation. *Harvard Journal of Law & Technology* 31 (2): 889–938.

Bell, B.S., A.M. Ryan, and D. Wiechmann. 2004. Justice expectations and applicant perceptions. *International Journal of Selection and Assessment* 12 (1–2): 24–38.

Bennett, A. 2019. Explainer—Deanna Amato's robo-debt case. Victoria Legal Aid. https://www.legalaid.vic.gov.au/about-us/news/explainer-deanna-amatos-robo-debt-case. Accessed 17 May 2021.

Berti-Equille, L., T. Dasu, and D. Srivastava. 2011. Discovery of complex glitch patterns: A novel approach to quantitative data cleaning. In *2011 IEEE 27th International Conference on Data Engineering*, 733–744. IEEE.

Carney, T. 2020. Artificial intelligence in welfare: Striking the vulnerability balance? *Monash University Law Review* 46 (2): 23–51. https://doi.org/10.26180/13370369.v2.

CEPEJ (Commission Européenne Pour l'Efficacité de la Justice). 2020a. European judicial systems - CEPEJ evaluation report - 2020a evaluation cycle (2018 data). https://www.coe.int/fr/web/cepej/special-file-publication-of-the-report-european-judicial-systems-cepej-evaluation-report-2020a-evaluation-cycle-2018-data-. Accessed 1 December 2021.

CEPEJ (Commission Européenne Pour l'Efficacité de la Justice). 2020b. CEPEJ tools on evaluation of judicial systems. https://www.coe.int/en/web/cepej/eval-tools. Accessed 25 November 2021.

CEPEJ (Commission Européenne Pour l'Efficacité de la Justice). 2020c. Mise en place éventuelle d'un mécanisme de certification des outils et services d'intelligence artificielle dans le domaine juridique et judiciaire, étude de faisabilité réalisée par la Commission européenne pour l'efficacité de la justice, 8 décembre 2020c, CEPEJ(2020c)15 Rev. https://rm.coe.int/etude-faisabilite-fr-cepej-2020-15/1680a0adf3. Accessed 4 March 2021.

Cerdeña, J.P., M.V. Plaisime, and J. Tsai. 2020. From race-based to race-conscious medicine: How anti-racist uprisings call us to act. *The Lancet* 396 (10257): 1125–1128.

Chadli, S., P. Neveux, and T. Real. 2021. Intelligence Artificielle et éthique: comment définir et mesurer l'équité algorithmique? https://www.quantmetry.com/blog/intelligence-artificielle-et-ethique-comment-definir-et-mesurer-lequite-algorithmique/. Accessed 25 November 2021.

Chereni, S., R.V. Sliuzas, and J. Flacke. 2020. An extended briefing and debriefing technique to enhance data quality in cross-national/language mixed-method research. *International Journal of Social Research Methodology* 23 (6): 661–675.

Coulon, J.M. 2008. *La dépénalisation de la vie des affaires: rapport au garde des sceaux, ministre de la justice*. La Documentation française. http://www.presse.justice.gouv.fr/art_pix/1_Rapport Coulon.pdf. Accessed 4 December 2022.

Croze, H. 2017. Justice prédictive: La factualisation du droit. *La semaine juridique-édition générale* 5: comm-101.

Delsol, J-P. 2021. Quand l'état de droit se fissure, la démocratie frissonne. *Les Echos* 3 Septembre 2021. https://www.lesechos.fr/idees-debats/cercle/opinion-quand-letat-de-droit-se-fis sure-la-democratie-frissonne-1343029. Accessed 25 November 2021.

Ellis, A. 2018. Neutrality and the civil service. In *Liberal Neutrality*, ed. Andrew Reeve and Robert E. Goodin, 92–113. New York: Routledge.

European Commission. 2021. The 2021 EU Justice Scoreboard. Communication from the Commission to the European Parliament, the Council, the European Central Bank, the European Economic and Social Committee and the Committee of the Regions COM(2021) 389. https://ec.europa.eu/info/sites/default/files/eu_justice_scoreboard_2021.pdf. Accessed 18 October 2021.

Fallery, B. 2019. Intelligence Artificielle: à qui profitent les ambiguïtés entre l'informatique, l'humain et la fiction? In *Journées IP&M sur L'Intelligence artificielle*. https://hal.archives-ouv ertes.fr/hal-03126061. Accessed 31 December 2021.

Ferrand, F. 2000. Le principe contradictoire et l'expertise en droit comparé européen. *Revue Internationale De Droit Comparé* 52 (2): 345–369.

Ferrand, F. 2015. L'offre de médiation en Europe : Morceaux choisis. *Revue Internationale De Droit Comparé* 67 (1): 45–84.

Gray, D. 2008. The people's courts? Summary justice and social relations in the city of London, c. 1760–1800. *Family & Community History* 11(1): 7–15.

Guggeis, M. 2020. The Responsibility of the European Legislator and of the National Parliaments for Improving Relations between European Citizens and EU Institutions. In *The crisis of confidence in legislation*, ed. Maria De Benedetto, Nicola Lupo, and Nicoletta Rangone, 259–284. Baden Baden: Nomos Verlagsgesellschaft mbH & Co. KG.

Hillebrandt, M., and S. Novak. 2016. 'Integration without transparency'? Reliance on the space to think in the European Council and Council. *Journal of European Integration* 38 (5): 527–540.

Hyde, A. 2019. Vers une cyber-éthique de la justice dite prédictive» Commentaire de la Charte éthique européenne d'utilisation de l'intelligence artificielle dans les systèmes judiciaires et leur environnement de la CEPEJ du 4 décembre 2018. *Dalloz IP/IT*. https://hal.archives-ouvertes.fr/hal-02395659. Accessed 31 December 2021.

Jaafari, M. 2016. Depenalization of business law. *The Judiciary Law Journal* 80 (94): 95–116.

Keyvanpour, M.R., M. Javideh, and M.R. Ebrahimi. 2011. Detecting and investigating crime by means of data mining: A general crime matching framework. *Procedia Computer Science* 3: 872–880.

Katz, P. S. 2014. Expert robot: Using artificial intelligence to assist judges in admitting scientific expert testimony. *Albany Law Journal of Science and Technology* 24(1).

Langford, M. 2020. Taming the digital leviathan: automated decision-making and international human rights. *AJIL Unbound* 114: 141–146. https://doi.org/10.1017/aju.2020.31.

Mateu, J., and J. Pluchart. 2019. L'économie de l'intelligence artificielle. *Revue D'économie Financière* 135: 257–272. https://doi.org/10.3917/ecofi.135.0257.

Maurel, L. 2019. Filtrage automatique et libertés: peut-on sortir d'un Internet centralisé? *Annales des Mines-Enjeux Numériques* 6.

Meunier, Axel, Donato Ricci, Dominique Cardon, and Maxime Crépel. 2019. Les glitchs, ces moments où les algorithmes tremblent. *Technique & Culture* 72: 200–203. https://doi.org/10. 4000/tc.12698.

Noriega, M. 2020. The application of artificial intelligence in police interrogations: An analysis addressing the proposed effect AI has on racial and gender bias, cooperation, and false confessions. *Futures* 117: 102510.

Ntoutsi, E., P. Fafalios, U. Gadiraju, V. Iosifidis, W. Nejdl, M.E. VidalS, F. Ruggieri, S. Turini, E. Papadopoulos, I. Krasanakis, K. Kompatsiaris, C. Kinder-Kurlanda, F. Wagner, M. Karimi, H.

Fernandez, B. Alani, T. Berendt, C. Kruegel, K. Heinze, G. Broelemann, T. Tiropanis. Kasneci, and S. Staab. 2020. Bias in data-driven artificial intelligence systems—An introductory survey. *Wiley Interdisciplinary Reviews: Data Mining and Knowledge Discovery* 10 (3): e1356.

Ogus, A. 1999. Competition between national legal systems: A contribution of economic analysis to comparative law. *International & Comparative Law Quarterly* 48 (2): 405–418.

O'Neil, C. 2016. *Weapons of math destruction: How big data increases inequality and threatens democracy*. New York: Crown.

Parviainen, J., A. Koski, and S. Torkkola. 2021. 'Building a Ship while Sailing It.' Epistemic Humility and the Temporality of Non-knowledge in Political Decision-making on COVID-19. *Social Epistemology* 35(3): 232–244.

Pasquale, F. 2019. A rule of persons, not machines: the limits of legal automation. *George Washington Law Review* 87(1).

Pasquale, F. 2020. *New Laws of Robotics*. Cambridge, Massachusetts: Harvard University Press.

Poizat, J.C. 2017. Nouvelles réflexions sur la «banalité du mal». Autour du livre de Hannah Arendt Eichmann à Jérusalem et de quelques malentendus persistants à son sujet. *Le Philosophoire* 2: 233–252.

Prakken, H., and G. Sartor. 2002. The role of logic in computational models of legal argument: a critical survey. *Computational logic: Logic programming and beyond* 342–381.

Queudot, M., and M. J. Meurs. 2018. Artificial intelligence and predictive justice: Limitations and perspectives. In *International Conference on Industrial, Engineering and Other Applications of Applied Intelligent Systems*, eds. M. Mouhoub, S. Sadaoui, O. Ait Mohamed, and M. Ali, 889–897. Cham: Springer. doi: https://doi.org/10.1007/978-3-319-92058-0_85.

Richard, C. 2018. Dans la boîte noire des algorithmes. *Revue Du Crieur* 3: 68–85.

Rigano, C. 2019. Using artificial intelligence to address criminal justice needs. *National Institute of Justice*. https://nij.ojp.gov/topics/articles/using-artificial-intelligence-address-criminal-justice-needs. Accessed 31 December 2021.

Ross, T. 1933. Machines that think. *Scientific American* 148 (4): 206–208.

Singh, Y., P.K. Bhatia, and O. Sangwan. 2007. A review of studies on machine learning techniques. *International Journal of Computer Science and Security* 1 (1): 70–84.

Singh, N., T.K. Bandyopadhyay, N. Sahoo, and K. Tiwari. 2021. Intellectual property issues in artificial intelligence: Specific reference to the service sector. *International Journal of Technological Learning, Innovation and Development* 13 (1): 82–100.

Spajosevic, D., A. Ittoo, L. Rebouh, and E. de Kerchove. 2020. *Study on the use of innovative technologies in the justice field*. European Commission. https://doi.org/10.2838/585101. Accessed 31 December 2021.

Stranieri, A., J. Zeleznikow, M. Gawler, and B. Lewis. 1999. A hybrid rule–neural approach for the automation of legal reasoning in the discretionary domain of family law in Australia. *Artificial Intelligence and Law* 7 (2): 153–183.

Stoett, P.J. 2019. *Global ecopolitics: Crisis, governance, and justice*. Toronto: University of Toronto Press.

T-540/15 Decision ECLI:EU:T:2018:167 22/03/2018 De Capitani/Parliament. https://curia.europa.eu/juris/document/document.jsf?text=space%2Bto%2Bthink&docid=200551&pageIndex=0&doclang=EN&mode=req&dir=&occ=first&part=1&cid=2072856#ctx1. Accessed 7 February 2021.

Thagard, P. 2004. Causal inference in legal decision making: Explanatory coherence vs. *Bayesian Networks*. *Applied Artificial Intelligence* 18 (3–4): 231–249.

Towell, N. 2017. Centrelink's robo-debt crisis: Who is Hank Jongen? *Canberra Times*. https://www.canberratimes.com.au/story/6037265/centrelinks-robo-debt-crisis-who-is-hank-jongen/. Accessed 10 November 2020.

Tung, K. 2019. AI, the internet of legal things, and lawyers. *Journal of Management Analytics* 6 (4): 390–403.

Ulenaers, J. 2020. The Impact of Artificial Intelligence on the Right to a Fair Trial: Towards a Robot Judge? *Asian Journal of Law and Economics* 11(2).

Wachter, S., B. Mittelstadt, and C. Russell. 2021. Why fairness cannot be automated: Bridging the gap between EU non-discrimination law and AI. *Computer Law & Security Review* 41: 105567.

Whittlestone, J., R. Nyrup, A. Alexandrova, K. Dihal, and S. Cave. 2019. Ethical and societal implications of algorithms, data, and artificial intelligence: a roadmap for research. *Nuffield Foundation.* https://www.nuffieldfoundation.org/about/publications/ethical-and-societal-implications-of-algorithms-data-and-articificial-intelligence-a-roadmap-for-research. Accessed 31 December 2021.

Chapter 15
Has the Case for the Case Been Made? Concluding Remarks

Dónal O'Mathúna and Ron Iphofen

Abstract This chapter brings together some of the general themes that can be gleaned from a consideration of all the case studies in this volume taken as a whole. Despite the substantive uniqueness of specific cases, no less than the ones collected here, there remain some key advantages to examining cases in detail and drawing on the broader lessons that can be learned from adopting the case study method. Equally important arc the lessons that can be learned about how ethically generated evidence can help inform trustworthy and effective policies.

Keywords Case study · Ethics · Case study method · Evidence

15.1 Where We Started

This volume set out to explore the ethical issues involved in research and other evidence-gathering activities in a way that encourages and supports policymakers in their use of 'ethical evidence.' This collection of case studies comes from the EU-funded PRO-RES Project which had as one of its aims to identify the various values, virtues, principles and standards that support the ethical practice of researchers, scientists, and, in fact, the diverse range of evidence-generators to be found in the modern world.[1] Another aim was to provide various resources that would assist those using research results and other evidence in making policy related to those topics. As discussed in Chap. 1, we believe case studies have a valuable role in

---

[1] PRO-RES is a European Commission-funded project aiming to *PROmote ethics and integrity in non-medical RESearch* by building a supported guidance framework for all non-medical sciences and humanities disciplines adopting social science methodologies. This project has received funding from the European Union's Horizon 2020 research and innovation programme under grant agreement No 788352.

D. O'Mathúna (✉)
College of Nursing and Center for Bioethics, The Ohio State University, Columbus, OH, USA
e-mail: omathuna.6@osu.edu

R. Iphofen
Independent Research Consultant, La Rochelle, France

© The Author(s) 2022
D. O'Mathúna and R. Iphofen (eds.), *Ethics, Integrity and Policymaking*, Research Ethics Forum 9, https://doi.org/10.1007/978-3-031-15746-2_15

helping policymakers reflect on existing policies and consider where policy should be changed or developed. Case studies are a significant element of the 'What Works' movement as a whole. The cases presented in this volume sought to show this value in a diverse range of areas addressed by non-medical sciences.

We believe that each of the case studies demonstrates particular ethical challenges being faced by researchers and those involved in various evidence-generating activities. Each case study explored challenges in various fields and disciplines that require ethical reflection that can contribute to appropriate policymaking in that area. The diversity of topics, fields and ethical issues are apparent from reviewing the Table of Contents. Part of the value of a case study is the detailed examination of a specific instance that it affords. At the same time, it is important to identify general principles and issues that can be usefully applied by policymakers more broadly. In this concluding chapter, we wish to pull together some of the general issues in and approaches to ethical evidence-based policymaking that are discussed in a number of the cases.

Six general issues are listed here and then will be discussed in more detail in the remaining sections.

- Research and policymaking as iterative processes
- The need for new policy
- The need for new cases
- Balancing principles
- Contextualization
- The value of cases.

15.2 Research and Policymaking as Iterative Processes

The ethics and integrity of research and evidence-generation have been the subject of much policymaking. This is explored in Chaps. 2 and 3 in regard to policies about Responsible Research and Innovation (RRI) and with data protection in Chap. 5. Beyond the specific policies themselves, these cases highlight the importance of policy itself becoming the subject of research. While RRI has been widely promoted and implemented, Chap. 2 discussed the results of some research which raised questions about how well understood RRI is, even by those who apparently fall under the requirements of that approach. RRI has been promoted in many parts of the world, and the case study in Chap. 3 discussed evidence of concerns about how culturally appropriate RRI is for low- and middle-income countries (LMIC), specifically India.

Chapter 5 presents the results of research exploring the impact of another major European Union policy, the General Data Protection Regulation (GDPR). This policy includes regulations about the appointment of Data Protection Officers which would sensibly appear to help support the implementation of the policy. However, the research discussed in this case study shows that simply introducing roles as part of policy is insufficient unless clear requirements for the role are included, and resources to support its activities are also provided. Without such support the role becomes supplementary and tokenistic.

In a different way, Chap. 4 affirms the value of evaluating and validating policy as it is being developed. The case study explored how the principles in the UK Association for Research Ethics Committees (AREC) framework were validated by the UK Office for Research Integrity (UKRIO) and the Association of Research Managers (ARMA) and how they confirmed their usefulness for the intended policy. The inclusion of this validation study during the policy's production helped not only to resolve disagreements during policymaking, but also helped to facilitate its acceptance when the policy was published. All too often research managers are neglected when research proposals are being assessed for the ethics entailed in their methodology, yet managers ought to be seen as essential to the dynamic nature of the research process.

We see in these cases that policymaking should include steps and plans to ensure that the policies themselves are subjected to research and other validation activities to ensure that they are based on evidence and to ensure that the impact of the policies is what was intended. If evidence is found that the policies are not achieving their aim, then changes and modifications should be made.

15.3 The Need for New Policy

The first general principle implies that policymaking is an on-going activity. As policies are evaluated, the need for change may be identified. The case study on wave power in Chap. 8 highlighted the need to ensure that policymaking is conducted with independence from those with vested interests in promoting or resisting specific policies. Chapter 13 explores how policies created prior to the COVID-19 pandemic were shown to be inadequate for the urgency of a pandemic. At the same time, various responses in research and public health showed the need for new policies to address the various practices and interventions proposed to respond to this emergency and others like it that are bound to emerge in the future.

A major focus within the PRO-RES project and also within this volume is related to emerging technologies. A new technology, such as artificial intelligence (Chaps. 13 and 14) or long duration space travel (Chap. 9) will require new policymaking. One of the themes in this volume that new ethical questions are arising for which we don't have answers or polices, and therefore more reflection, analysis and policy are needed. But this is not only for novel technologies. Chapter 12 examines a case study in *One Health* where the novelty arises from research and practice bringing different disciplines together. The isolated ethical issues related to humans, animals or the environment are not new, but what is new is the way *One Health* research requires the balancing of these different disciplines in ways that neither researchers nor policymakers might have foreseen.

Policymaking should be seen as an iterative process, where new technologies, new circumstances and new collaborations will require careful reflection on the adequacy of existing policy and a commitment to revise what needs to change and to engage with the making of new policy when gaps are identified.

15.4 The Need for New Cases

Another general finding is that innovative research is constantly leading to the need for new case studies. As research continues to explore new areas and topics, to develop new devices and abilities, and to generate new questions, ethical issues will be raised that themselves need to be explored and then policy designed to address them. Case studies have an important role to play in exploring these innovations and challenges. This was seen with research that takes humans deeper into space (Chap. 9) or as AI is applied in legal and law enforcement settings (Chap. 14).

New cases to assist the exploration of emerging technologies and innovations can usefully come from other fields. Historical examples of technologies which at the time were new provide useful case studies because they show how their novelty was addressed at that time. Those lessons can help policymakers as they address today's (and tomorrow's) new technologies. The value of such case studies was shown in Chap. 7 where the superconductor case continues to shed light on publication ethics, and in Chap. 8 where the wave power case highlights the need to address conflicts of interest.

New cases are not only related to technology, but also to social practices and research methods themselves. The case study of urban explorers (Chap. 11) raises issues about new developments in research methods, here focused on the development of autoethnography and the paradigm shift from researchers taking objective and impassive, neutral stances to one where researchers are subjectively immersed in the research and impact directly what happens. While some would see the virtue of 'courage' entailed in some research engagements, the nuances and complexities that a case study reveals points to its long-standing value in understanding the ethical challenges of conducting 'disruptive' research.

Such new areas of research and technology bring challenges because of the uncertainty and lack of information upon which to base decisions and policies. The space exploration example highlights issues for all "first in human" experiments—no one knows exactly what will happen. How then can policymakers be evidence-based when the evidence is lacking or non-existent? The standard ethical approach to addressing risk has been to allow people to make informed decisions. Yet that is not possible when there is little evidence with which to inform participants. As Chap. 9 discusses, the next best thing may be to encourage transparency about the information that is available. For policymakers, transparency will be important about how any standards and guidelines are developed and the decision-making principles used in setting those standards. Uncertainty was also a factor raised with AI during the COVID-19 pandemic (Chap. 13). The reliability and relevance of the data available, and its insufficient quantity, all led to questions about the efficacy of the technology. Uncertainty does not only exist in regard to the technology, but also to those impacted by its application. Hence, the uncertain basis for AI generates concerns about its variable impacts on different populations, communities, and groups, particularly given the potential for those who are already vulnerable to being more negatively impacted by the technology (Chap. 14). Again, openness and transparency came up in several case studies to address such dilemmas.

15.5 Balancing Principles

Promoting evidence-based policymaking when evidence is lacking is just one of the dilemmas raised in this volume. A common feature in many of the cases was how researchers and policymakers can be required to balance different ethical principles in what are often impossible dilemmas. With wave power (Chap. 8), transparency in decision-making had to be balanced against government strategic requirements for security. With superconductors (Chap. 7), the push to publish for the sake of open science competed with the need for secrecy to ensure financial gain. In the Belfast Project (Chap. 10) balancing research participants' confidentiality and safety appeared to conflict with the importance of criminal justice; protecting the rights of those who participated in violent struggle with the rights of victims for answers, truth, and justice. As the Belfast case noted, it can be argued that the requirements of the criminal justice system should always take precedence over ethical issues in research, yet the conundrums revealed in this and other cases can instead point to the need for new policies and ways to address the dilemmas themselves.

Covert research leads to another difficult balance (Chap. 11). Here, the value of informed consent and how it respects participants' autonomy can come into conflict with the potential benefit that may come from research. However, this particular case raises further complexity in balancing the role of researchers as impartial observers versus active participants. Also difficult here is the importance of the research data and the issues explored, particularly as it sheds light on the needs and issues of actual people as opposed to the legality or otherwise of the practices themselves.

Such issues raise particularly challenging dilemmas for policymakers as now they must decide if they will use the results of research which itself broke policies and/or laws while being conducted. Much as some researchers have argued that researchers who violate research ethics principles or codes during their research undermine the credibility of the research enterprise and bring its stakeholders into disrepute, policymakers who use research of questionable origins risk undermining the very purpose of their discipline and practice. What is at stake is the need to strike a balance that best promotes all of the ethical principles that are in conflict, even if no proposal promotes all principles completely. Chapter 13 concludes with a list of policy recommendations on how to balance conflicting principles, in this case regarding urgency and benefit in the COVID-19 context.

15.6 Contextualization

Our introduction (Chap. 1) raised the importance of context and discussed how case studies help to make its role transparent. This came up clearly in Chap. 3 in the discussion of RRI in India. Context was discussed here at both the conceptual level, and in terms of policy implementation. Another important aspect of this is how different contexts can shed important light on a policy which ultimately benefits multiple contexts. Here, the Indian concept of Scientific Temper can bring new insight to RRI that can take it beyond its European focus as initially conceptualized and developed. Another approach to contextualization is revealed in Chap. 6 where the case study examined the International Network for Government Science Advice (INGSA). The way INGSA has organised itself around regional chapters allows geographical concerns and approaches to be addressed in different ways without insisting on one global approach to research ethics or the understanding of ethical evidence.

Contextualization also applies to timing, in the way the COVID-19 pandemic impacts the cases in Chaps. 12 and 13. This brings in the need for flexibility in policy, as has happened with innovation in the research ethics practices and policies during the pandemic.

15.7 The Value of Cases

Case studies provide a way for those who participated in historical situations to share their experiences in ways that can benefit others, including policymakers. The cases about ARMA (Chap. 4) and wave power (Chap. 8) take this approach. This is one way that lessons can be learned which take account of how the case actually happened. Such cases are, necessarily, provided from the perspective of those involved, as opposed to that of a dispassionate researcher or uninvolved observer. While that carries some risk of bias being introduced, this can be acknowledged explicitly and at the same time allow for lessons to be learned.

Other case studies were written by those who were not directly involved and allow lessons to be learned from past examples (Chaps. 3, 7, 10 and 11). The depth given provides a way for policymakers to learn from past practices and see whether some or all aspects of the case could be implemented elsewhere or at a different time. The evidence from one case study does not suggest that this is the best way for policy to be made, but at the same time can provide more details about why things were done and what may be useful as policies are developed elsewhere. Drawing from such historical case studies allows the articulation of principles to guide policymakers, such as was done in Chap. 4 for principles that should underlly policies for ethics review. Other policymakers can then apply such principles elsewhere in the development of their policies.

The process of producing policy, particularly policy regarding research ethics, should follow the same principles that the policy expects of researchers. In other words, if policymakers expect researchers to uphold certain principles regarding ethics and evidence in the conduct of research, then equivalent principles should be upheld during the policymaking process. Chapter 4 articulates four ethical principles for researchers (independence, competence, facilitation, and transparency) holding that three of these apply directly to policymakers in their work (independence, competence, and transparency).

The educational role of case studies is demonstrated very transparently in the superconductor case study (Chap. 7). As each aspect of the historical case is explored, questions are put to readers encouraging them to use the PRO-RES toolbox to reflect on the ethical questions raised and how an ethics tool can be used to stimulate reflection on a complex and challenging case. In keeping with many of the other cases explored in this volume, simple answers are not available and for some questions the most that can be provided is a call for further reflection, discussion, and evaluation. Such is the nature of the ethical challenges faced by researchers and those seeking to develop policies related to research.

15.8   Conclusion

All evidence gatherers and users, be they researchers, research managers, funders, civil servants, journalists or politicians, know that research can never be a 'pure' activity; it can never be fully divorced from special interests, ideology, methodological preferences and simple prejudices. Researchers should strive to ensure such influences do not excessively detract from the ambition of the research engagement to produce something of value, something that matters, something that helps direct policy to be both efficient, effective and honest. It is in this 'striving' that research can become 'objective' and ethical. It is in the detailed study of specific cases that we can demonstrate how difficult this is to achieve and yet how such difficulties can be addressed or even overcome. In these case studies we have seen the challenges that have to be faced in remaining ethical and some of the ways in which such challenges have been resolved. The details help us see what can be done, what has been done and, crucially, often what we should have done to ensure evidence is gathered in the 'right' way.

Index

© The Editor(s) (if applicable) and The Author(s) 2022
D. O'Mathúna and R. Iphofen (eds.), *Ethics, Integrity and Policymaking*, Research Ethics Forum 9, https://doi.org/10.1007/978-3-031-15746-2

Printed in the United States
by Baker & Taylor Publisher Services